Natural Healing
for Babies
and Children

Natural Healing for Babies and Children

Aviva Jill Romm

The Crossing Press
Freedom, California

The information contained in this book is based on the experience and research of the author. It is not intended as a substitute for consulting with your physician or other health care provider. Any attempt to diagnose and treat an illness should be done under the direction of a health care professional. The publisher does not advocate the use of any particular health care protocol, but believes that the information in this book should be available to the public. The publisher and author are not responsible for any adverse effects or consequences resulting from the use of any of the suggestions, preparations, or procedures discussed in this book. Should the reader have any questions concerning the appropriateness of any procedure or preparation mentioned, the author and publisher strongly suggest consulting a professional health care advisor.

Library of Congress Cataloging-in-Publication Data

Romm, Aviva Jill.
    Natural healing for babies and children / Aviva Jill Romm.
        p. cm.
    Includes bibliographical references and index.
    ISBN 0-89594-786-2
    1. Pediatrics—Popular works.   2. Children—Diseases—Alternative treatment.   3. Naturopathy.   4. Herbs—Therapeutic use.   I. Title.
RJ61.R72 1996
618.92—dc20   95-50884
                                                              CIP

ACKNOWLEDGMENTS

My deepest appreciation goes to my children, Iyah, Yemima, Forest, and Naomi, who have taught me step by step how to care, listen, nurture, and play; who have been patient with me when I've been less than patient with them; and who have given me opportunities to learn about health and illness.

Wordless gratitude goes to my mate, Tracy Romm, who has been the "first among equals" in my life, especially during the many hours it has taken to produce this book. I love you.

Deep appreciation to my mom, Wendy Perlman, for encouraging and tolerating my love of words, and to my grandma Ida, for feeding me in many ways.

Heartfelt thankfulness goes to my friends, colleagues, and teachers: Sarahn and RaAum Henderson, Lisa Olka, Nzingha Alkebu-Ian, Lizzie McDaniels Feigenbaum, Eve Coppedge-Waldron, Jeannine Parvati Baker, and Frank Trocco, all of whom at various times encouraged and supported my writing, my vision, my family, and my soul.

Thanks also to Debbie Pulley, Claudia Conn, Dr. Dayle Hawthorn, Kim Land (for the last-minute computer rescue), and the many midwives, herbalists, and physicians who have always been willing to share their knowledge and experience, and to the many families who over the years have given me the opportunity to see natural healing at work.

I am very grateful to Dr. Vance Dietz for providing a thorough medical review of this book, Halim Provo-Thompson for initial enthusiasm and endorsement, and to Elaine Gill, publisher; Linda Gunnarson, editor; Fran Haselsteiner, copy editor; and the fine staff at The Crossing Press, for helping me make this book the finest it could be. And, finally, my deep thanks to the plants themselves, for sharing their healing whenever called upon.

Contents

Foreword

Natural Healing for Babies and Children drives home one of the most natural principles of health care: the more informed are the parents, the healthier are their children. With this book, Aviva Romm encourages parents to be active participants, rather than passive recipients, in the health care of their children and gives parents the tools to take responsibility for health care decisions.

Traditional medicine, while necessary and lifesaving in many circumstances, often ignores the mind-body connection and the miraculous ability of the body to heal itself—given the right boost from nature's natural medicines. The information in this text is meant to be in addition to, not a substitute for, your child's doctor. It makes parents *partners* in the health care of their family, helping them use common sense remedies and good nutrition to improve the health and well-being of their children.

This is a timely book. The inevitable health care "reform" will be a mixed blessing. On the one hand, parents will have less access to doctors to heal their children. On the other hand, the beneficial effect of this change is that people will have to take more self-responsibility for their health care. They will have to rely more on nonprescription health care products, and one of these will be herbs.

Parents must become experts on their children. No one else will. Throughout this book the author recommends a high-touch style of child care, which I call "attachment parenting." This way of caring for babies and children helps parents get to know their child, to be more sensitive to the well child, and therefore to know more intuitively how to treat the sick child. I applaud the author for presenting the health benefits of massage, good nutrition, and breast-feeding.

The body has a tremendous capacity for healing itself, yet sometimes we have to help it along a bit—naturally.

—William Sears, M.D.

Introduction

This book was created for parents who want to care for their children in ways that are natural, safe, affordable, and environmentally conscious. It offers herbal and other natural remedies that speak to our desire to improve and maintain the health of our families, prevent illness, and feel capable of caring for ourselves.

Conventional medicine is a mixed blessing. It best serves our needs in crises that require heroic intervention. Blood tests, antibiotics, and any number of medical procedures allow us to gain sometimes-essential information and even save lives. But modern medicine also gives us the feeling that health care is something "done to us"—that we are passive, not active, participants in our own health. This can be very disempowering.

People who feel disempowered generally fall into one of two categories. One type seeks professional care for every complaint, ending up with overtreatment, overmedication, and to top it off, an overpriced doctor's bill. The other type avoids medical care by ignoring a problem and hoping the symptoms will go away. As a result, these people may wind up with a more serious complaint that might have been resolved readily at the onset, or they may live with chronic discomfort affecting the quality of their lives. The first type believes that illness is insidious and that our health is fragile and dependent on the medical profession. The second type avoids doctors for financial reasons or out of a real fear of being subjected to unnecessary procedures and treatments that physicians often employ in order to cover themselves in the event of litigation.

This book represents a balance between the extremes. By using it to explore the nature of the illnesses and discomforts that commonly affect your children, you can learn when home care is reasonable and how to do it, and when to seek help without giving up your sense of involvement and empowerment. You will learn practical, traditional methods of improving, maintaining, and restoring your children's well-being. By becoming more of a participant in your own wellness and that of your children, your confidence will grow and so will your relationship with those you care for.

For the past thirteen years, in order to care for myself, my husband, and our four children, as well as those who come to me for midwifery care or herbal information, I have been researching and exploring the practice of natural healing. The term *natural healing*, to some degree, could refer to all healing modalities that exist, because humans are part of nature and, by extension, all we "create" is technically part of nature as well. When I refer to *natural healing*, however, I am specifically talking about methods and remedies that generally fall outside the realm of conventional medicine, including herbalism, nutritional awareness, homeopathy, and massage. Natural healing also involves an awareness of the connection between mind and body and the ways in which that relationship influences our health. The remedies utilized in natural healing are not synthetic; they require little mechanical processing; and because they may be purchased without medical prescriptions, they are easily accessible. Even more than the actual substance or technique used, natural healing is based on the premise that our bodies are wisely designed to maintain health, and that given nourishment and support when needed, they will do so. It is, one could say, an approach to medicine based on confidence in the perfection and logic of the body. This view differs from that of conventional medicine, which considers the body a machine that cannot maintain adequate functioning without regular trips to the repair shop, the doctor being the mechanic.

Because we lack the extended community common to previous generations, this book is intended as a companion for parents, linking us all in an extended network of families committed to the well-being of children. This network is global. I believe that we can all support one another and reclaim our ability to care for ourselves through traditional, natural remedies if we pick up the threads of the old ways where modern technology took over and combine the best of both worlds. Traditional Chinese medicine has a term for this. It is called "walking on two legs."

In the spirit of those who came before us, this book is a collection of knowledge, beliefs, and customs to be handed down for the benefit of the next generations. Its roots are multicultural, ancient, and contemporary. It embraces both the unwritten and the well documented. May this offering be a nourishing fruit for you and your family, and may it contain within it seeds to plant in the hearts of others.

How to Use This Book

- Browse through the book from front to back, or however you like, to get a general idea of the contents. Ideally, you might read the book through once to familiarize yourself with the approaches and techniques before you need them. That way, when you need information quickly, you'll know where it is and have on hand the supplies you are likely to need.
- Feel free to really *use* your copy. Make notes near things that work and don't work for you; jot down new things you learn.
- Approach this information with the spirit of adventure. The techniques and remedies described stem from a variety of experiences— my own and those of other midwives, parents, and herbalists, as well as from well-documented research. Not all remedies are effective or appropriate for all people at all times. By trying a wide variety of natural approaches and keeping notes of what you use, you can help add to the data base of natural health information.
- Always heed the precautions listed with herbs or conditions, and consult with an experienced health care practitioner when necessary.
- Many of the formulas in this book are equally effective for adults, but not all of the preparations are safe for use during pregnancy. Pregnant women should therefore do further research or consult with an experienced herbalist before self-prescribing herbal remedies.

PART I

HERBALISM
AND
NATURAL HEALING

Chapter 1

❖

Toward a Deeper
Understanding of Health

We live in what is considered a "health-conscious" society: People jog
and do aerobics, watch their weight and fat consumption, take vitamins
and eat high-fiber cereals. Yet heart disease is still a major cause of death;
obesity among children and adults is on the rise while anorexic teenage
girls are starving themselves.

The problem is that our "health consciousness" is not really that at
all, but rather a quest for the "perfect body" or a daily life free of illness
so we can work more, stay up later, stay young longer. We have mistakenly bought into the idea that health is a certain kind of body or lifestyle,
not an intrinsic sense of strength and wellness. Our standards of health
are based on external ideas—the size of the clothing we wear; how long
we can sustain our heart rates while jumping around in Lycra tights; how
much we look like that tall, thin, white, twenty-two-year-old fashion
model in the television commercial. As long as we continue to search
outside ourselves for a standard of what health "looks like," we won't
succeed, because some of us are short; some are black, yellow, or brown;
some of us are stocky; and some of us ride around in wheelchairs.

What we need to do is redefine our standard of health so that it is
based upon our own individual sense of well-being.

❖ REDEFINING WELLNESS ❖

Learning to be aware of how we feel as part of our early life education
and learning basic health skills enable us to do things that help us feel
well and truly love who we are. This may involve dietary awareness,
exercise habits, or the ability to stand up and demand one's right to a
healthy environment. It may mean learning to live in good relationship
to one another. It may take on transpersonal meaning as we commit to
ensuring health for all humanity. In this aspect, health may mean giving
and sharing so that all can have enough. As a culture this means ensuring decent housing, meaningful work, and high-quality foods for all of
our members because a desire to live and the ability to enjoy life are at

the heart of health. Without hope for the future, the human organism has no need to maintain vitality and, therefore, health.

Health is not the absence of disease. It is an inner spark that glows from the core of a person outward. As a culture we have adopted a materialistic concept of health and illness. We address the complaints of the body as mere physical symptoms and attempt cures that attend only to these physical manifestations of disease. But health can have as much to do with our emotional states, our immediate surroundings, and our levels of harmony with the natural world. For example, when parents call me about a child with chronic earaches, I will gently ask whether they have been arguing within the child's earshot. Almost invariably this query will lead to a discussion about the stress they've been having in their home. Children are incredibly sensitive to subtle energy, and their illnesses are often, though not always, a reflection of their environments or their efforts to cope with stress.

Our approach to healing can incorporate awareness of the more subtle spiritual, mental, and emotional aspects of life and the ways these can become disturbed, resulting in physical illness. All of human life comes down to forces that no science or technology can explain. Modern medicine is just beginning to acknowledge—as evidenced by research into the efficacy of such techniques as biofeedback for reduction of hypertension and acupuncture for pain relief and drug addictions, as well as studies confirming that constant stress is detrimental to one's health—what traditional cultures all over the world have recognized: that not all of life can be reduced to a purely measurable, physical understanding or explanation.

Cultures around the world look to nature and to the psyche of the person in need for a deeper understanding of illness and healing. For example, practitioners of Ayurvedic medicine (a two-thousand-year-old healing system well developed in India) sometimes prescribe fairy tales as part of a medical treatment, the idea being that the messages revealed in the stories will help the person unlock mental patterns that may be the source of the problem. A Native American may go to a shaman who will fast and pray to particular nature spirits or deities with whom the patient is perceived to be in disharmony. Healing the disharmony between the person and the environment is seen as necessary for the improvement of physical illnesses.

In our own culture, we have come to see the body as a fragmented series of parts and ourselves as separate and distinct from our surroundings. Illness becomes merely the action of germs in our bodies, and the impact of our personal lives and lifestyles are treated as insignificant.

Perhaps this is why the most common complaint about medical care is that it is impersonal, that people are treated as test results, or worse yet, like automobiles on an assembly line. A person's life is not considered a significant factor in wellness or illness.

In our daily lives, most of us are somewhat divorced from the rhythms of the natural world. We go to sleep late, eat processed and refrigerated foods, spend much of our time indoors, and regulate our environment with thermostats. In many ways we've become "soft." As our lifestyles move farther away from daily interaction and harmony with natural cycles, we lose not only our instinctive ability to recognize what we need for health and healing, but our bodies also come to forget what health really is. We merely adapt to a second-rate level of wellness, one in which headaches, constipation, ear infections, hemorrhoids, and backaches are accepted as normal complaints. With just a little effort we can change these patterns. Through small acts performed each day—taking a moment to breathe deeply, looking at the nighttime sky, "sitting in our bodies"—we can learn to remember how intrinsically healthy we are.

❖ TEACHING OUR CHILDREN ABOUT WELLNESS ❖

As parents, we have the opportunity to show children how intimately their personal health is connected to their surroundings. This is a very important teaching on many levels because it enables children to value themselves and to see the importance of creating surroundings that support them. This has many personal, social, political, and environmental implications. When we teach children that illness is something to avoid at all costs and to overcome as quickly as possible regardless of the means of doing so, we deny them the right to take time to heal, honor their illnesses, convalesce, and grow. We are denying that illness is a natural part of health, and we make them enemies of their bodies. As herbalist Lorien Cruden says, "The way you care for your child's health teaches them positive or negative body images: wholeness or alienation."

We can give the very best health insurance to our children: We can help them learn to care for themselves early in life by helping them live closely to nature, teaching them to eat well, exercise often in the fresh air, and have a positive attitude toward life, health, and their bodies. We can teach them to recognize when a situation is causing stress and how to handle it. We can teach them to recognize and respond to early signs of not feeling well, and to take care before they become sick.

The word *nourish* appears many times in these pages, so a definition is in order. The words *nutrition* and *nourish* have their roots in a verb meaning "to suckle." Another related word, *nurture*, means "affectionate care and attention." *Nurture* is also defined as "the sum of the influences modifying the expression of the genetic potentialities of an organism."

So we see that nourishment is much more than obtaining a certain amount of vitamins and minerals from food. It is also a way of loving and caring for ourselves and others that stimulates the unfolding of our greatest skills, health, and humanity—our genetic potentialities. Physical nourishment in the form of food is required, of course, but so are exercise and rest as well as attention to the complex emotional and psychological needs of human beings.

In providing care, nourishment, and attention to young children, we give them permission to grow into self-loving, self-nourishing adults. If we introduce children at a young age to a way of life that encompasses natural elements, this consciousness will remain a part of their identities and sense of what is important. Helping children accept themselves from a young age will decrease the incidence of anorexia among teenage girls, reduce the peer pressure that often results in drug use, and foster human beings who are accepting of others. We will have raised a generation of people who resist the building of toxic dumps in their neighborhoods (and, perhaps, in all neighborhoods, not just their own), the use of chemicals in their foods, and even intolerable work conditions. In short, attention to health becomes a whole life issue, not just a prescription for herbs or vitamins.

❖ TEACHING OUR CHILDREN ABOUT HEALTH RESPONSIBILITY ❖

The notion of preventing illness does not mean that we must avoid illness at all costs. Being a fanatic about health is just the opposite extreme of not taking any responsibility at all, and it doesn't teach kids to feel relaxed about themselves. If we think we must live "purely" and do everything "perfectly" to conquer or escape illness, we are creating the inner stress of always fighting or avoiding something. This is an illusion that creates an enormous amount of performance pressure, limits us from experiencing and enjoying life, and inevitably leads to disappointment or frustration when illness does arise. The goal is not to arm ourselves against illness. What we are trying to do is avoid unnecessary or repeated illnesses that come from lack of nourishment, which can include a lack of healthy foods, insufficient rest and relaxation, inadequate exercise, and even a lack of warmth and caring from others in our lives. And, when illness does occur, it can be as much our goal to attend to it with grace and hope as it is to prevent it.

Remember, there is no one, pure perfect path. Occasional illness or even serious disease can be experienced within the context of health. Life experienced through the fear of illness and death is not life at all but a grand avoidance. When we begin to accept ourselves, even with our illnesses and weaknesses, we begin to give ourselves unconditional love. When our children become ill, they know that it is just part of life, not the result of anything they have done wrong. There is no need for guilt or embarrassment. Ultimately, health is loving ourselves "for better or for worse." This is the place from which true healing occurs and is a way of life worth passing on to our children.

Health requires, as Lorien Cruden puts it, "participation in life." We take responsibility for our well-being and our environment on all levels—physically, mentally, emotionally, and spiritually. We don't wait for someone to come and fix us; we don't give up our power and responsibility because of fear. We put ourselves into nourishing situations because we deserve to feel well.

❖ Empowering Our Children ❖

We want our children to trust their bodies' ability to maintain and restore balance and health, we want them to understand the simple ways that help maintain health and remedy illnesses, and we also want them to grow up feeling empowered and in charge of their health care, rather than vulnerable or victimized at the times they require medical assistance.

Perhaps the most significant teaching tool available to us is our example. Making it a priority to care for our own wellness and doing the things that promote our health, we give our children encouragement to do the same. We are providing a model that says, "I value my body and my health." In addition, when ill, if we modify our lifestyles and give attention to restoring our wellness, we are giving our children a valuable demonstration of personal responsibility.

How we interact with and allow ourselves to be treated by health care workers is also important. Through this example we teach children that we are passive recipients and victims of health "care," or that we are active participants, in fact organizers, of our health care. When we enter a doctor's office, for example, do we get our questions answered, our fears addressed, and, in general, feel that we got what we paid for? Did we feel in command of the visit, or did we feel intimidated by the doctor-patient interaction? We need to feel strong and confident in a doctor's office, not threatened and meek. We need to ask our questions until we are satisfied with our understanding of the situation, and, above all, recognize that we are paying the physician to serve us, rather than the physician doing us a favor by allowing us a few minutes of his or her time. If we cower, then we teach our children to cower; if we are confident, we give a special gift to our kids.

If a family's health care decisions are made by one person (for example, mother, father, or doctor) without the consent or feedback of the one receiving the care or treatment, a child may come to see health care as something that happens to someone rather than something one plays a central role in. It is essential that our children feel able to express what they are feeling both about their bodies and in response to their health care needs and recommendations, and that they are able to influence what happens to them.

By this same token, they can, from an early age, be given understandable explanations about their bodies when they ask questions or are experiencing something they don't understand. In this way they learn not only about bodily functions, but also how to gather information, an essential skill for being able to take responsibility in many areas of life. As we explain health conditions to them, should they arise, we can explain treatments and remedies, educating them as well as providing a rationale for what we are suggesting they need, and eliciting their cooperation.

It is important that we help our children value their bodies as strong, reliable, and resilient. If we are overprotective and give remedies for every small complaint, we eventually give our children the message that they are frail and that their bodies depend on external means to be healthy. When herbal remedies, drugs, or other treatments are needed, they can be presented with language that reflects our respect for the body's healing powers. For example, a child with a cold can be told that "extra sleep will help your body heal this cold" rather than "sleep will cure your cold," or "these herbs will help your body heal this cold" rather than "these herbs will cure your cold." Emphasis is placed on the body, not the treatment, giving the child the message that the body is fundamentally responsible for health.

As we nurture a generation of educated and empowered individuals, we are sowing seeds of change toward a healing network of mutual participants rather than a health care system that is a hierarchy of providers and recipients.

My children enjoy taking walks to search for and gather plants for use in our home. One daughter will talk to and caress a plant the way she would a kitten. When they are ill, they know to take a relaxing bath, drink tea, dress cozily, and snuggle in bed or be massaged, read, or sung to. When we use herbs, they are used as loving nourishment. The teas are caring made physical. Our children's bodies can readily heal themselves; the plants are a supportive rather than an attacking method of healing.

Meanwhile, over the years, our children have seen us learning to overcome our fears. They have seen us wonder if we are doing the right things for them, they've seen us panic and seen us ready to attack any "invading" illness, and they've seen our doubts while we were learning to trust that our bodies can heal and that nature is our greatest healer. Through it all they have seen us learn and grow to levels of awareness beyond our doubts—and this is also a healing they get to witness.

Each day we practice that health care is not something that is done to us, that it is not something that victimizes us. Sometimes when our children have been ill we have, out of fear, battled with them to "take their remedies" ("Take your medicine!" "Eat your vegetables!" Sound familiar?). Our children continually remind us that everything is working as it should, in its own time. When we step back in quiet observation and let the illness unfold while we support the child with comfort and gentle, simple remedies, we have better results and happier children. This does not mean that strong and unpleasant herbs are not sometimes necessary; however, we can enlist our children's participation in taking their remedies through encouragement and positive motivation rather than making them feel victimized.

Everyone has fears and doubts. These can feel overwhelming when we are taking the great responsibility of caring for our children's health, especially if our choices are criticized by others. Feelings are powerful teachers and guides that we should listen to, not ignore. We can learn more about ourselves by identifying our feelings and fears and by watching how they influence our actions. Beneath feelings of fear we can learn to identify our inner voice and use this to reach deeper levels of self-trust and understanding. This inner voice is often felt as a physical feeling at the gut level. It is a feeling that almost seems to say yes or no. We can use our inner voice to help us determine whether our fear is an anxiety-based reaction or an inner message warning us of danger, and then determine the most appropriate responses.

There is so much that we as parents can do to care for our children at home naturally and gently, and so little required to do it—just the willingness to educate ourselves about natural healing techniques and home health care, to cultivate our powers of observation, and to learn to trust our judgments and decisions. These are ongoing processes. What we learn will continue to serve as tools that our children can use for a lifetime and, in turn, their children as well. Of course, the time you invest in educating yourself will be rewarding in very practical ways—for example, your kids will spend less time being ill and your family will have lower medical expenses. But let us remember that true health is more than not getting sick or having an athlete's body. True health means possessing a good feeling about oneself and an ability to approach life with a zestful attitude. It is a feeling of powerfulness about one's life. This is what we can give to our children as we also explore the world of natural remedies.

Chapter 2

❖

Herbal Medicine

Since the beginning of time, people worldwide have relied on plants and other natural materials for maintaining and restoring health. Nearly every culture has a rich herbal lore and broad repertoire of remedies for conditions that commonly affect its people. Many of these traditions, such as traditional Chinese medicine and India's Ayurvedic medicine, have been extremely well developed and well documented for thousands of years. Other systems, such as those indigenous to Africa and the rainforests of South America, are no less sophisticated but have remained undocumented because their societies lack written traditions. Nevertheless, these cultures have informed us of some of the major medicines used in our society. For example, quinine, used in the treatment of malaria, came from the bark of *cinchona,* or Peruvian bark, found in South America, as did wild yam (*Dioscorea villosa*), from which we derive some streroids and birth control pills. A plant now being studied is the Madagascar periwinkle (*Vinca rosa*), from which a promising anti-tumor substance has been extracted. We know about these because native peoples employing these plants for medicinal purposes have shared their knowledge with ethnobotanists.

European culture also has a rich tradition of herbalism. In fact, many European herbs are the foundation of modern pharmaceutical preparations. Unfortunately, during the Middle Ages, herbalists, most of whom were women ("old wives") were prosecuted for the alleged practice of witchcraft and much of our common herbal knowledge was lost or legally proclaimed the domain of doctors. In modern Europe, however, there has been a resurgence in the acceptance of herbalism and homeopathy, as well as new interest in other herbal traditions such as Chinese medicine.

In the United States, natural healing has been obscured by an element of distrust and unacceptance, in large part because of the American medical system's influence. Historically, since the 1800s, "regular" doctors, those with some formal training in medicine, have tried to debunk the credibility of traditional healers. In reality, traditional healers, or lay practitioners, had significantly more training and clinical experience than the regulars. Medical training in the nineteenth century often was no longer than two months long and offered little, if any, clinical experience. In addition, lay practitioners used gentler remedies and treatments, far safer than their counterparts use of substances like mercury and sulfur used as internal remedies and blood-letting, used as an external treatment for diseases sometimes as mild as regular headaches. The Popular Health Movement, a lay health movement of the 1800s, primarily an early feminist organization, was trying to educate the general public about the importance of hygiene, good nutrition, fresh air and exercise, and comfortable clothing for women. By 1910, a report by the Carnegie Foundation, known as the "Flexner Report," gave public acclaim and financial support only to those institutions that would train practitioners as regular doctors and discredited all other medical institutions, eventually causing them to close. The Popular Health Movement eventually fell by the wayside. Currently, those schools endowed by the "Flexner Report" are still at the forefront of medical training. Examples are Harvard Medical School and Johns Hopkins University. The regular doctors now hold a near-monopoly on the health care profession.

This veil of suspicion is still evident in the many states where such arts as midwifery, acupuncture, and herbalism are illegal and medical doctors who use unconventional healing modalities in their practices are subject to ridicule and legal harassment from their colleagues. Slowly, however, natural healing approaches are again becoming more visible to the public, more viable as an option in health care.

❖ Why Use Herbs? ❖

People have used herbs to heal illnesses for centuries. But today, pharmaceutical medications for nearly every medical condition are available. And most of these drugs are simple to take: a pill or sweet-flavored syrup, even a single injection that can last for months. Usually no preparation is required of the purchaser. So why would anyone want to use herbs?

An herb is a plant that was a vital and intact being, drawing nourishment directly from the earth and the elements. When an herb is respectfully harvested, most of its essential properties and vital essence are retained. Within each herb is a perfect mixture of various chemical substances—sugars, alkaloids, and minerals, for example. In most plants these substances balance and buffer one another so that an herbal tea does not contain pure alkaloids, for instance; the mixture of chemical components present in herbs usually mitigates the effects of their stronger chemical constituents. While some plants are deadly poisonous if ingested in even small amounts in their natural form, the majority of herbs are remarkably safe.

Pharmaceutical drugs are a different matter. While many drugs were originally derived from plants, the final preparations that reach the consumer are no longer in their naturally occurring forms and combinations. The medicine we take usually is an extract of the chief or active ingredients, commonly the alkaloids, the most potent and potentially dangerous chemical substances in the plants. Ingested in concentrated form, without the buffering action of other ingredients, these drugs can easily be harmful.

Most drugs today are synthetic substances, meaning that they are not the direct and naturally occurring extracts of plants but laboratory-created simulations of the original chemicals. Few synthetic drugs have been tested over time. In fact, many drugs on the market have not been proven fully safe for human consumption or given full approval by the U.S. Food and Drug Administration (FDA). This is especially true in the case of drugs used throughout the childbearing cycle and for young children. According to Dr. Donna Kraus, a pharmacologist at the University of Illinois in Chicago and author of the textbook *A Pediatric Dosage Handbook*, anywhere between 60 and 80 percent of the prescription drugs sold in the United States are not approved for use by children. Drugs approved for use by adults are commonly given to children even though they are not necessarily tested and proven safe for such use and even though proper dosage guidelines are not established for them. (These statistics are derived from the September 1994 issue of the *Annals of Pharmacotherapy*, and a December 1994 issue of the *Wall Street Journal*. The articles are titled, respectively, "The Need for Conducting Research on Medications Unlabeled for Use in Pediatric Patients," by Nahata, and "F.D.A. to Make It Easier for Drug Makers to Give Pediatric Data to Doctors," by Kessler.)

Two infamous examples of synthetic drugs that have been widely used without full knowledge of their potential hazards are diethylstilbestrol (DES) and thalidomide. DES, a synthetic form of estrogen, though never proven safe in laboratory animals in the 1930s, was by 1942 still being given to women with FDA approval to women to prevent lactation and to treat menopausal symptoms and vaginitis. By 1947 the FDA approved its use for pregnant women with histories of miscarriage, high blood pressure, and even slight bleeding in pregnancy. Although by 1953 DES had been conclusively proven ineffective in the prevention of miscarriage, the FDA did not denounce its use in pregnancy until 1971. By that time its connection to cancer in users and children of those who had used it during pregnancy was becoming well documented. DES and similar hormones are still used today in many countries for lactation suppression, acne treatment, morning-after contraception, and other applications.

Thalidomide, a sedative drug prescribed to pregnant women in Europe in the 1960s, is another of many examples in which use of a synthetic drug had disastrous side effects. Thousands of babies born to mothers who took thalidomide were severely deformed. Though the drug had a number of critics before its introduction, thalidomide was pulled off the market only when the scale of the problem became evident.

While pharmaceutical companies are able to sell inadequately tested substances for general consumption, the FDA regularly removes from the market herbs that have been safely used for generations. Some herbs, such as comfrey, are alleged to be carcinogenic (cancer causing). But research usually studies effects of concentrated extracts of a plant, not the whole plant. If you were to extract oxalic acid from spinach and test its safety by administering high doses to laboratory rabbits, you would find it to be poisonous. But does that mean that spinach, eaten in moderation as a vegetable, is harmful? Of course not. So it is with herbs. We must look at the effects of the whole plant, not just highly potentized extracts.

Another advantage of herbal remedies over newly "discovered" and synthetic drugs, especially for minor health concerns, is their long-term use. In a sense they have been proven safe historically. Of course, herbs can also be used as drugs and can have serious side effects, but centuries of clinical trials have yielded a wealth of information proving the general safety and efficacy of many herbal remedies. A large and continually growing body of scientific knowledge substantiates this empirical knowledge. Medications come and go from the drug market, but people have been using the same plants for thousands of years.

The development of new medications is extremely expensive, involving research and development, advanced laboratory technology, testing, advertising, packaging, and a host of specialists to carry out these steps. The pharmaceutical industry is a huge, profit-oriented enterprise. In a 1990 personal interview with the author, Dr. James Duke, at the time a leading economic botanist for the U.S. Department of Agriculture and author of many books and papers on plant medicines, estimated that it costs an average of $231 million to prove a new drug is safe and efficacious, noting that "our drug companies don't want to prove herbs safe and efficacious because you and I would be out there self-medicating and they wouldn't get their $231 million back." Because so many drugs require a physician's prescription, and therefore an office visit, the price to the consumer goes up dramatically. By contrast, herbs are inexpensive, even free when you harvest them from the wild or grow them yourself.

Natural remedies allow one to use preparations that are not only beneficial for the individual but also ecologically responsible, an important consideration for the present and the future of planetary health. Harvesting herbs and other natural remedies with an awareness of plant habitat and availability (avoiding endangered plant species, of course) is significantly less harmful to the environment than medicines made from rare plants that are then synthesized from petroleum-based products and other hazardous or scarce substances. In fact, in most aboriginal cultures, the health of the individual and the health of the surrounding ecosystem are recognized as inseparable. The practice of natural healing helps us restore our own connection with the natural world.

Traditional healing methods—those passed from generation to generation, among friends and neighbors and between cultures—have been with us for as long as our existence on our planet. Although we who live in highly industrialized societies may not be familiar with these ways, people all around the world still rely extensively upon herbs and common-sense practices as their main medicines. In fact, the U.N. World Health Organization (WHO) has recognized the importance of herbs and traditional remedies: They are readily available, affordable, reliable and effective; and when used appropriately they have few, if any, negative side effects. The WHO has been making international efforts to train local indigenous healers and to encourage people to preserve and make use of their traditional healing systems and medicinal plants.

This brings us to another important reason for using herbal medicine: personal empowerment. We live in a society in which health care is as much an economic and a legal issue as it is one of human caring and health. From the insurance companies to the hospitals to the doctors there is money to be made in health care. The high cost of medical care is partly justified by the expensive training, equipment, and procedures it requires, the costs of which are recovered by charging steep prices. It is true enough that doctors are a hard-working, dedicated lot, but doctors also have incomes that are substantially higher than those of other hard-working and important members of society. (Have you ever considered what our health would be like if we had no sanitation workers?)

How is it that we let ourselves pay such a high price without saying "Enough!"? The answer is vulnerability. We feel so ignorant about our own bodies that we are dependent on experts for information about ourselves. Of course, there will always be times when an experienced voice will be necessary. But as a society we have abdicated our responsibility for ourselves and left it up to medical professionals to tell us what to do. The medical profession's near-monopoly on health care reinforces the belief that this is the correct approach. Yet when the outcome is not to our liking, we blame the very ones we went to for guidance; we sue the doctors! Ironically, our litigious approach to medical care perpetuates patterns of overtreatment and overprescribing as physicians attempt to protect themselves from accusations that they didn't "do everything they could."

Both medical professionals and health care recipients are caught in a vicious cycle. The most promising way to break this cycle is to take responsibility for our own health and that of our families. When we educate ourselves by reading, by attending classes and workshops with experienced practitioners, and when we practice home health care, we gain a depth of knowledge and insight that guides us in making appropriate choices, thereby enabling us to take more control of our health. If, as a society, we take this responsibility, we will find the power and confidence to demand decent medical care at fair prices. We will have the freedom to choose the forms of care, whether they are "conventional" or "alternative," that we feel best serve our needs. As we become confident that it is possible to be our own experts, we will feel less vulnerable and we will lessen our dependence on the health care system. Physicians may realize that they depend on us for jobs perhaps more than we depend on them for our health. As we gain empowerment from promoting our health, we may also begin to take greater control of other areas in our lives where we feel vulnerable, ignorant, or taken advantage of. Taking charge of our lives may be more important than we realize. According to Alfie Kohn (1993), "research has found that people who rarely become ill despite having to deal with considerable stress tend to be those who feel more control over what happens to them."

The history of medicine reveals the depth of antagonism exhibited by sanctioned medical professionals toward traditional healers and their skepticism about traditional healing modalities. Healing does not, however, have to be the domain of any specific philosophy. It can be all inclusive, as is currently being shown in Europe, where most medical professionals accept the idea of "complementary medicine," which recognizes the value of using natural medicines in conjunction with appropriately applied allopathic treatment when needed. While medicine in Europe is still governed by agencies designed to license practitioners, complementary medicine represents a step in a better direction: a health care system offering a multiplicity of options. In a system of medical choice, people have the right to choose options that best suit their needs, including their health care providers, even if they choose themselves to fulfill their primary health care needs. As empowered and educated people, we are capable of making such choices responsibly.

❖ Working with Herbs ❖

Modern Western medicine is based on the germ theory, which considers disease to be the result of pathogenic organisms invading the body, and healing to be based on the elimination of such organisms. Symptoms are discomforts to be suppressed. All of this is accomplished with medications that may in the long term have damaging effects upon the body. When symptoms are suppressed, the body is unable to alert us to illness. The very medications designed to kill invading organisms may in the process injure our own healthy organisms and natural defense systems.

Herbalism sees us as capable of healing ourselves given the elements needed for health: trust in our own "vital force" (our inherent body wisdom that guides us toward life and health), and foods, herbs, and care that enable the body to perform its functions unhindered. While antiviral or antibacterial herbs may be used, the general approach is not one of "attack and destroy" but "support and nourish." Nature is given the upper hand because we trust that the Earth's plants are endowed with the right properties our bodies need for health. Herbalism draws on the concept of *ecoevolution*—that is, all species, including humans and plants, continue to evolve in response to similar environmental factors.

Though herbs can be used in health crises and emergencies in conjunction with conventional medical treatment, "an ounce of prevention is worth a pound of cure." Providing care that strengthens the child in the absence of illness—excellent nutrition, hygiene, and attention to overall health—is easier than trying to fix a problem after it arises. Likewise, attending to small symptoms when you notice them, is better than ignoring them and giving them the chance to develop into large problems.

It is essential to know the effects of the herbs you are using and respect their strength. Some herbs are very strong and need to be used in small quantities. Through studying books and using mild herbal remedies you can discover the benefits of many herbs and learn if they have side effects or contraindications. (Of course, you should read about all herbs *before you use them*. You must know about possible side effects before you use any medications, including natural ones.) Proper dosage is very important.

Start by working with mild herbs in small dosages. Often that is all you need. You can always increase the strength of a remedy. Remember that you are augmenting the body's natural tendency toward well-being; you need not attack or overpower with herbs. A gentle and consistent approach works best. Always keep in mind the unique needs of the person taking the herbs, adjusting dosages according to age and weight. Use all your senses to assess whether certain herbs are appropriate for the individual. If possible, try remedies on yourself and feel how they affect you before giving them to someone else.

To be most effective, a sufficient amount of an herbal remedy needs to be consumed. Ideally, the remedy can be taken in small, frequent doses throughout the day, giving the body a steady amount over a period of time, thereby allowing not only the physical substances of the plant a chance to act, but also allowing the more subtle energies of the herbs to fill the patient. It is as if each time you drink, eat, or otherwise work with an herb, you are inviting the plant to work with you for your healing. Herbs can work whether you "believe" in them or not, but you can enhance healing by creating a positive mental state for the recipient of the remedies. Psychological attitude is well acknowledged to be an important factor in recovering from even major illnesses.

A word is necessary here about the time required for herbal healing. I've seen herbs work quickly many times, but usually herbal therapies are slower acting than synthetic preparations. A person treating a simple infection with an antibiotic can return to normal activities in just a few days, continuing the medication on the job or at school. A person choosing to heal an infection with herbal remedies must be patient, giving the treatment a chance to be effective. While one can take herbs when at work or at school, the general approach of natural healing is to allow for healing to be a gentle process; it does not rapidly force the body back into balance so one can immediately resume normal routines. I firmly feel that this is healthier for the human organism in the long run, but it does require a commitment of time and a willingness to prepare and take the herbal remedies.

❖ HERBAL MEDICINE FOR CHILDREN ❖

Using herbs with children is particularly easy. A child's metabolism is quickly responsive to most substances, and it is with children that plant medicines are quickly and noticeably effective. In an age when our environment is facing incredible crises, introducing children to the wonderful world of plants is a way to foster their respect for the Earth and a lifelong commitment to caring for it.

Taking time with your child (or self) during illness is a requisite for healing. One herbalist states that when she tries to cope with her child's illnesses in a peripheral fashion, attitudes are poor and healing is prolonged. When she turns her full attention to the child, he responds more quickly on all levels, and she has a better experience, too.

Pharmaceutical drugs require only peripheral attention to a child's illness. Of course, a parent can and should give focused care to a child whether or not pharmaceuticals are in use, making any illness a bonding experience for both. To use herbal remedies with your child, you need to develop both knowledge and experience. You must judge for yourself what you are capable of and confident in handling. It is also wise to join a supportive network of people already knowledgeable in natural health care who are willing to assist you when you have questions or require further resources.

An excellent way to develop your confidence with herbs is to begin using them in simple health and minor first-aid situations, like colds, headaches, small cuts, and minor burns. As you read the chapters in this book that describe herbal remedies for specific conditions, keep in mind that each child is unique and may require an individually tailored remedy. If one formula doesn't seem to be working for you or your child, try another. As you gain a sense of each plant's individual "personality" as well what your child needs, you will develop a sense of which remedies will likely give you the results you want.

Often, as people begin to reclaim the responsibility for their own health care, they are tempted to do it all for themselves. This is not only unnecessary, it is impossible; we are all interdependent beings. For example, you may have a great deal of knowledge about woodworking, but if you were trying to build your own house and ran into an unfamiliar situation, you would be wise to seek the advice of someone more experienced. So too with natural health care.

In many instances, simply a more accurate diagnosis can be just the information we need to successfully heal ourselves or our children. Sometimes a different approach is helpful or necessary. Nor should we consider ourselves failures if we need to rely upon standard medical care or pharmaceutical preparations. There is a time and place for just about everything, and it is wise to have humility. Natural healing does not mean rejecting other forms of help. It is an inclusive approach.

If you put some time and commitment into learning how to use natural remedies for yourself and your children, you will open many doors for yourself. You will see that you can become very knowledgeable about health care; you will gain a deeper appreciation of the beauty and wisdom in the natural world; and you will find yourself becoming even closer to your kids. Be patient, and one day you will realize just how much you have learned. And the exciting thing is that there are always amazing new things to learn about plants and about our health.

Chapter 3

❖

Home Health Care for Children

In learning to care for your child's health, the best knowledge you can acquire is the insight you gain from becoming closer to your child. When you spend a great deal of time together, you become keenly aware of your child's subtle ways of being. You will quickly recognize when your child is "not acting quite right." Early signs of illness become obvious to you. You can then offer your child the special care and nourishment that prevent a small bit of not feeling well from turning into a major illness. Major illnesses rarely come out of nowhere, and accidents are also more likely to occur when a child is ill, tired, or otherwise "off balance." Early awareness of illness allows you to care for the child with milder methods and herbs than is possible with more advanced conditions.

You can also learn to recognize the signs and symptoms of childhood illnesses. You may want to purchase a pediatric reference book at a medical or used bookstore or some of the books listed in "Further Reading."

Developing your resources and abilities takes time, but keep in mind that most children do not have life-threatening illnesses and accidents, so you need only general knowledge. A course in cardiopulmonary resuscitation (CPR) is valuable for anyone who spends a lot of time with children. Consider starting a study group where you live: You are bound to find other parents like yourself who want to learn more and take greater responsibility for the wellness of their families.

❖ THE BASIC PHYSICAL EXAMINATION ❖

Knowing what is generally considered "normal" physical health and development in children can help develop your confidence in assessing your child's wellness. Remember, all children are different—"normal" is just a *general range* that healthy children usually fall within. Each child has his or her own variations of normal. If your child seems healthy, she likely *is* healthy. Major variations from the norm may be cause for further exploration. Any variations from your child's own typical well-being are certainly cause for further exploration as they may signal an illness. Pay close attention when you notice changes during or after a trauma or an illness.

Dr. George Wootan, an advocate of home health care and creator of the weekend intensive training course called "Pediatrics for Parents" (see "Resources") and the book *Take Charge of Your Child's Health,* recommends in his classes that parents give their children general physical exams at home on a regular basis until their bodies become familiar. This suggestion may be worthwhile to follow as you are learning to practice home health care. It gives you a regular time (once a month is sufficient) to check your child's physical health while sharing some time together. Keep dated records in a small notebook: basic physical statistics (height, weight, heart rate, and so forth) and any significant milestones, developmental steps, illnesses, and treatments, as well as any cute, witty, or otherwise charming things your child has recently said or done. You can even include a current photograph of your child. This little book will be a warm memento of childhood that you can present as a gift when your child is grown, and of course it serves as a comprehensive health history.

Once you realize that you are familiar with your child's unique body and behavior, you can discontinue your routine checkups and do them only when you feel they are needed. However, you may discover that you enjoy the time spent with your child and want to continue with body awareness games (which can be found in the yoga and exercise books for children in "Further Reading") and massage (see below) as part of an overall approach to health care.

To do a basic physical exam, not much different from what you might be paying a pediatrician to do, you can simply give your child a "once-over" as you give him a bath or help him get dressed, noting whether anything seems unusual. You can also turn it into a game. Let your child give you an exam, too. The idea is to get to know your child, not perform a prodding or peering exam. You can learn how to check heart and respiratory rates, pulse, and temperature, all of which most children find fun and fascinating. Older children will naturally be beyond the stage when a silly approach is appropriate, but they can be taught to recognize what constitutes good health and what symptoms they might feel if an illness is coming on (see "Common Early Signs of Illness" later in this chapter). You can teach older children about basic anatomy and physiology by listening to your hearts and lungs, and looking at each other's eyes or even ears if you have an otoscope. This is an excellent opportunity to teach children about hygiene, nutrition, or whatever personal or general health topics arise.

Giving your child a massage on a regular basis is another caring way to stay in touch with and promote your child's physical well-being. Massage usually is welcomed by younger and older children alike. You needn't be a professional massage therapist to give a simple neck-and-shoulder rub or a back-and-foot rub. A book on massage for children, such as *Infant Massage*, by Vimala Schneider McClure (which also has sections on massaging older boys and girls), will be very useful as you learn.

The following information is intended to give general guidelines for recognizing normal ranges of "vital signs" and health in kids. Always remember that these are just averages and that every child is unique. Various factors can influence and alter these signs. For example, exercise and excitement, as well as nervousness, increases pulse and respiratory rates. Temperature is higher in the afternoon than in the morning by as much as a whole degree. For more detailed instruction on doing a basic physical exam, see the books *A Parent's Guide to Childhood Symptoms*, by Dr. Richard Martin; *Taking Charge of Your Child's Health*, by Dr. George Wootan; and *A Guide to the Physical Examination*, by Dr. Barbara Bates.

While the overall procedures for examining babies and children are similar, babies are given specific attention in Chapter 6, "Your Healthy Newborn." The following is geared toward young children (ages one to six) and older kids (over six). These guidelines do not give you the ability to diagnose every symptom that your child might have, nor should you use this approach to look for problems. But spending this time with your child will enhance your relationship, and you'll be more aware of situations when your child seems subtly out of balance. In turn, you'll know when to provide him or her with extra support and prevent illnesses from becoming serious. Early prevention is always preferable to treating advanced problems. You may, in the case of simple problems, refer to this book or others for treatment suggestions, or you may need to consult a doctor.

A few basic supplies are helpful to have for exams: a penlight, a tape measure, a scale (regular bathroom type), a stethoscope, a watch with a second hand, a notebook, and a pen. Parents who want to learn to examine the ear canal and eardrum may want an otoscope. The stethoscope is not absolutely necessary because you can place your ear on your child's chest to hear heart and lung sounds, but it is helpful for hearing clearly, and with it your child can hear his own heart and lungs. Reasonably priced stethoscopes are available from Cascade Health Care Products (see "Resources").

Let your exam be casual. It can take place on your child's bed, in the living room, wherever both of you are comfortable. It can be a private affair or a family activity. Begin by asking your child (if she is old enough to answer you) specific questions about how she is feeling. If she is ill, ask whether she has any pain or discomfort, and if so, let her show you where. Inquire whether any of her friends, teachers, or others she has been with recently are ill. Ask your child what she thinks the problem might be. As much as we know our children, they know themselves even better. Let them take part in their own health care. Empowerment can begin at an early age.

General Appearance

Observing your child's general appearance is the logical way to begin your physical exam. It should be done casually, preferably without your child knowing it, so you can see her natural posture and behavior. Note how your child moves, sits, or stands. Does she seem upright or slouched? Comfortable or uncomfortable? Listen and observe how she speaks. Is her tone of voice pleasant or whining, normal or loud? These are important signs because, for example, a child who is very whiny and speaking loudly may simply be tired or may have an earache that is affecting her temperament and hearing (which will affect speech). For other general signs to look for, see "Common Early Signs of Illness," later in this chapter.

The Skin

Your child should be fully unclothed (of course, underwear is fine for older or modest kids) so you can see the whole body. Take note of the size, shape, and texture of any "birthmarks," moles, lumps, or other markings. These are not uncommon, and you need only watch for changes, such as darkening and growth in size or number.

Look at cuts for cleanliness and healing. Notice the presence of bruises, boils, or a rash. The latter two could indicate infection or allergy.

Pay attention to whether the skin feels moist or dry, warm or cold. Also notice the skin's color. Yellow skin could indicate jaundice and possible hepatitis; pallor could indicate a recent fright or anemia; redness could be caused by a fever, and blueness could indicate respiratory or cardiac problems.

The Head

Generally feel and look over the head to check for lumps, dry scalp, and ticks or lice if your child has been exposed to either. If your child has headaches, ask where they are and how they feel. Look at the child's head for symmetry as well as proportion to the body. In very young kids the head may seem slightly large, but this is the normal way the body grows. Brain development and head size occur at a slightly faster rate than the body, but by four years old, everything looks proportional. The hair should have some bounce and shine if nutritional needs are being met. Rate of hair growth and hair thickness are individual matters.

THE EARS

The ears are a common site of infection in children and therefore worry for parents. Because of the proximity of the ear canal to the back of the throat and sinuses the ear is a place where fluids can pool and bacteria can thrive. To watch for problems, you can purchase an otoscope, a tool for examining the eardrum, through a medical supply company or through Cascade Health Care Products (see "Resources"). Otoscopes can run anywhere from $20 to $400. Ask a friendly health care professional to teach you how to use it, or refer to one of the books mentioned earlier.

The healthy ear canal is pink and contains some ear wax. You need not remove ear wax unless it is interfering with your child's hearing. When necessary you can use ear candles (ask at a local health-food store) or an ear syringe (available at any pharmacy), but these measures are rarely needed. Tenderness, redness, pus, or drainage in the ear canal is a sign of inflammation or infection and should be treated. The normal eardrum (tympanic membrane) appears as a transparent or opaque disk through which you can see the bone called the hammer (malleus). An eardrum that appears bulging, inflamed, cloudy, or yellowish (from pus) indicates an ear infection. A perforation in the drum or drainage coming from it indicates that the eardrum has ruptured. You can recognize an ear infection when you have a clear idea of how a healthy ear looks, so look at your friends' and family members' ears whenever you get the chance.

Look behind the ears for cuts, skin problems, and health of the skin.

You can check your child's hearing with games. Whisper something to your child from varying distances, or hold a ticking watch close to the child's ear and slowly move it farther away (an inch or so at a time), taking note of how far away your child is still able to hear the sound. A hearing problem may simply be due to fluid congestion in the ears but should be evaluated if it persists beyond a few weeks, if it develops suddenly after a high fever, or if it occurs in the complete absence of a head cold.

THE EYES

When you look directly at your child, notice whether his eyes seem clear and sparkly or red and dull. Dull eyes may be a result of fatigue, allergy, or oncoming illness. Sties, discharge, itching, or swelling occur with allergies and infections. Dark circles under the eyes, also known as "allergic shiners," may come from a food or environmental allergy if your child is generally well rested (they are also associated with fatigue). The eyes should neither bulge (thyroid problems) nor be sunken (dehydration). The eyes and the lids should be basically symmetrical, the pupils about equal in size, and the pupils equally responsive to light. To check for this, have your child look at your penlight and notice the contraction of the pupils. Then turn off the light—the pupils should dilate. Since difference in the size of the pupils after a head injury can indicate serious head damage, pupils equal in size are important to identify.

Vision can be checked with a basic eye chart. Or play a game: have your child read street signs or spot small landmarks at a distance. Does your child squint? But remember that your child may not know what you are pointing to, so don't assume that not "seeing" it indicates vision problems.

THE NOSE

See if there is any nasal discharge. Clear or whitish discharge may be from a cold or allergy, whereas yellowish or greenish discharge results from upper respiratory and sinus infections. Tenderness along the sides of the nose and over the sinuses also indicates sinus infection. A foul-smelling discharge could occur if a foreign object is lodged in the nostril. Have your child gently blow or sneeze it out. If it is quite stuck or it is something that would have become swollen, such as a raisin, take your child to a physician for help in removing the object. Do not try to force it out.

THE MOUTH AND THROAT

Have your child open her mouth wide and stick out her tongue as far as possible (the proverbial "Aaaaahhh" sometimes helps). Using your penlight, look at the back of the throat. The throat, tonsils, and uvula (the structure in the center that hangs down from the back of the throat) should be pink. Redness and swelling indicate infection. The tonsils, which are glands, may swell when the body is resisting an infection. Pus or white spots indicate infections (for example, strep throat or the measles), and white patches in the mouth that can't be easily removed are often from thrush (an oral yeast infection).

Examine the tongue for sores; notice whether the breath is generally pleasant or not.

Check the gums and teeth for general health. Gums should be pink, shouldn't bleed after brushing, and should not exhibit sores. The teeth in young children are very white; permanent teeth are slightly less white and shiny. Brown spots, either stains or cavities, should be looked at by a dentist for optimal cavity prevention. Daily dental hygiene including brushing at least twice a day and daily flossing will prevent decay in most children. (If you took certain antibiotics, such as tetracycline, during pregnancy, the child may have stained teeth.)

THE NECK

Have your child move his neck in a full range of motion. While a child may have an occasional stiff or sore neck, as from sleeping in an awkward position, movement should be pretty easy and painless. Stiff neck accompanied by fever is an important diagnostic sign of meningitis. If your child is ill and can't place his chin to his chest without pain, seek medical help immediately. Meningitis is life threatening.

The neck has many lymph nodes. In most adults they are not visible to the eye, but in children, you can sometimes see lymph nodes when they turn their heads from side to side. This is normal as long as the nodes are not swollen. Of course, you must know how they feel normally to know if they are swollen. So when your child is well, check out the lymph nodes in the neck. "Swollen glands" is just another way of saying "swollen lymph nodes." Lymph nodes that remain persistently swollen, hard, or red, or which grow in size in the absence of a head or chest cold, need further assessment by an experienced practitioner.

THE CHEST AND LUNGS

Listening to the lungs with a good stethoscope is not difficult. (You can usually find one for $20 or less at pharmacies, or you can purchase one through Cascade Health Care Products; see "Resources.") You do not have the same breadth of experience as a physician who listens to thousands of chests, but you can familiarize yourself with your own children's normal lung sounds and respiratory rates. At minimum this is fun and interesting for your children. The lungs should sound clear; you should easily hear air reaching different points on the chest over the lung area. During a cold you will hear rattly, mucousy sounds. Painful breathing accompanied by fever may indicate pneumonia, which warrants immediate medical assistance.

To find the rate of respiration, count the number of breaths you hear in sixty seconds (look at your watch). Respiratory rate is affected by activity level, but the normal range is as follows: 30 to 80 beats per minute in a newborn, 20 to 40 during early childhood, and 15 to 25 during late childhood. The adult level, about 12, is reached by age fifteen.

Look at the chest and under the armpits for swollen lymph nodes or any unusual characteristics. Breast-fed babies as well as pubertal girls and boys may exhibit swollen tissue. The swelling will usually resolve itself (of course, pubertal girls are developing breast tissue).

The Heart

Normal heart rates in children are as follows:

1 to 2 years	110 beats per minute
2 to 6 years	103 beats per minute
6 to 10 years	95 beats per minute
10 to 14 years	85 beats per minute

To listen to the child's heart rate, place your stethoscope (or your ear) over the left breast, and count the beats you hear (a "lub-lub" counts as one beat) for sixty seconds as you look at your watch. Heart rate varies some from child to child. Activity levels, relaxation levels, and fevers also alter heart rate. Fever will increase heart rate by about 10 beats for every degree of temperature over normal.

You are not likely to gain the experience to detect heart abnormalities by listening to your child's heartbeat. If your child's skin episodically turns blue (cyanosis), a serious heart problem may be the cause; contact your physician or medical center.

The pulse can be felt on the thumb side of the wrist. It corresponds to the heartbeat. A child who has been very active or who has an infection has an elevated pulse. In Chinese medical diagnosis, the pulse is felt in three different sites on each wrist, and at three depths, revealing a great deal of information about the functioning of the organs and overall health. For our purposes, we can feel whether the pulse is strong or weak. A healthy child will have a pulse that feels firm and steady but is not pounding.

The Abdomen

Young children normally have protruding bellies. When the child is four to five years of age, the belly becomes more proportional to the rest of the body. A belly that suddenly becomes bloated could indicate intestinal parasites or a bowel obstruction and requires further evaluation.

Since children are often ticklish, you will need to move your hands slowly and gently over the abdomen. Talk with the child to distract her from feeling ticklish. You can give your child a belly massage with a nice herbal oil, all the while taking visual note of any findings and feeling for lumps or unusual places. A lump at the navel is probably an umbilical hernia, most of which spontaneously resolve by the end of early childhood. Severe abdominal pain, either independent of touch or occurring when you press an area of your child's abdomen, requires medical attention.

The Genitals

If your child's genitals appeared normal at his or her first examination (which you or your spouse, midwife, or doctor performed shorty after birth), chances are he or she is still perfectly normal. As you bathe your kids, help them get dressed, or see them nude, just notice whether everything looks fine. The penis should not be unusually red at the tip, nor should there be any discharge in either boys or girls. Occasionally, however, the child may have a small amount of a creamy substance in the labia or beneath the foreskin. This can simply be washed off in a bath. Uncircumcised boys, after about three years old, may develop a buildup of this substance (smegma), which can become infected, so teach them to wash gently beneath the foreskin with each bath (at least twice weekly, more in warmer weather and as they get older).

Teenagers begin to go through many physical changes usually around age twelve or thirteen. Some kids mature earlier, others later. Remember that emotional changes will be occurring, too, and many of the child's needs, including his or her nutritional requirements, will change. An excellent book for both parents and teens is *Changing Bodies, Changing Lives* by Ruth Bell.

Close in proximity to the genitals is the anus. A red anus may indicate a food allergy, while itching may be due to an allergy or to pinworms. Healthy elimination is important, but what constitutes health is an individual matter. Regularity is going to be your biggest clue. Your child may poop twice a day or once every two days, which could still be considered normal. Very hard or very loose stools mean that you may need to modify your child's diet or he may be becoming ill. Frequency of urination is also an individual matter, depending on kidney and bladder health, amount of fluids consumed, and the age of the child. Any sudden increase could indicate a urinary tract infection. Sudden decrease could mean inadequate fluid intake, dehydration, or a kidney problem.

I hope these guidelines help you to become familiar with what is normal for your child and realize that you are in the best position to know this. As you spend time learning about your child's health, your ability to make use of this information will grow, and you will feel increasingly confident in evaluating when home treatment seems advisable and when you need to seek medical care.

❖ COMMON EARLY SIGNS OF ILLNESS ❖

If your child exhibits any of the following signs, she or he may be becoming ill:

- Changes in eating habits
- Behavioral changes (crankiness, irritability, lethargy, fatigue, uncooperativeness, drowsiness, sleep disturbances)

- Complaints (sore throat, swollen glands, headache, runny nose, stomach ache)
- Pain
- Chills, fever, quick pulse (or unusually slow pulse), respiratory changes
- Bowel and urinary changes (frequency, color, odor, consistency)
- Skin changes (temperature, color, moistness, rashes, sensitivity such as itching)
- Ears hurt, hearing seems "off "
- Eyes watery, glassy; circles under eyes
- Dizziness, clumsiness
- Vomiting
- Coated tongue
- Disinterested in play (This may be one of the most significant changes we notice.)
- Voice changes (hoarseness, whining)

If any of these occur, it is the perfect time for some herbal teas, the choice and quantity appropriate to how the child feels. It is also a time for extra rest, attention, and perhaps changes in diet. These steps can offset the illness or at least minimize your child's discomfort and the length of the illness. Of course, if you see many symptoms or your child seems seriously ill, seek medical care promptly.

Since illnesses that are caught early are the easiest to treat, try to trust those little inklings that tell you your child feels "off." You don't have to feel that you're being overprotective, and your child may just appreciate that extra bit of attention.

❖ THE SIX STEPS OF HEALING ❖

The main concern of parents working with home health care is how far they can go with it: What can be handled at home given their skill and what they have around the house, and how serious the situation. I would like to share with you an approach to healing taught to me by Wise Woman herbalist Susun S. Weed and shared here with her consent. Known as the "Six Steps of Healing," this system can assist you in choosing the appropriate response to your child's health care needs. These steps are applicable in an infinite variety of circumstances and are offered as guidelines for the various decisions you may face regarding what treatment to use an when. The following are Susun's steps with my interpretations.

Step 0: Do nothing to interfere; observe. Recognize and observe the processes taking place. Allow the processes to unfold. Sleep, meditate, rest.

Step 1: Gather information. Refer to books, consult support groups, use low-tech diagnosis (such as visual assessment, Chinese pulse diagnosis, and noninvasive physical exams), divination, and intuition.

Step 2: Work with the energy. This may be in the form of Bach flower essences, color healing, homeopathy, prayer, visualization, ritual, music, laughter (or crying), brightening up a room, opening windows.

Step 3: Nourish and tonify. Use herbs gently as food and nourishment. Physical activity, lifestyle changes, massage, baths, etc., can all support and comfort your child. The work of nourishment is immediate (as in a good meal or a hug); tonification (use of herbal tonics or regular massage, for example) requires repetition because it works by bringing about gradual beneficial changes.

Step 4: Stimulate or sedate. Use herbs as stronger medicines. Acupuncture, remedial massage, and hot and cold water treatments also fall within this category. In this step you are becoming more assertive in your approach.

Step 5: Use supplements and (pharmaceutical) drugs. Use synthesized or concentrated compounds such as vitamin supplements and medications. Supplements can often be given without prescriptions, but as with medications, excesses can have serious side effects and cause harm. Antibiotics and all other nonherbal medicines are in this category.

Step 6: Physically invade. Use invasive diagnostic tests including x-rays and other internal examinations, colonics, or surgery. This step includes any procedure that requires physical entrance into the body in a forceful way. Susun includes fear-inspiring language in this category; for example, you're ready to take your newborn home from the hospital eight hours after birth, and a pediatrician tells you that newborns are prone to infection and can easily become deathly sick in a matter of hours, so you should stay at the hospital for an extra day while tests are run to make sure your (visibly healthy) baby is okay.

Knowing your child well is the best knowledge you can have. If you combine that knowledge with the above guidelines for healing, and trust in your own judgment, you have a lot to go on. Observation along with presence of mind and courage are worthwhile skills to develop and practice if you are planning to implement home health care. I do not believe that anxiety has ever healed an illness, but your sense of peace can help your child relax and get on with the work of healing.

Although not a "step" per se, any and all actions you take should be preceded and accompanied by observation. Look at and try to recognize the processes taking place. Do nothing to interfere; allow the processes to unfold. Continue your careful watch even if you have found yourself going through all the steps. In fact, after each step you take, it is important to reevaluate the situation.

Let's apply the steps to a practical example. You notice that your child has a slightly runny nose with no other symptoms. Your first response may be to do nothing except continue observing the child. You may see the runny nose as a minor inconvenience or even as a "clearing out" and just let the child's body do its thing without further assistance. You may, however, based on other observations, see that the child is coming into a full-blown cold, in which case you decide to work with the energy (Step 2) by making sure that the environment is warm and comfortable, that the child's clothing is comfortable and of a pleasant color, and that your home is calm. You may also prepare light and nourishing teas and foods and help your child get to bed early, letting her whole being be nourished by sleep (Step 3, "Nourish and tonify"). If you don't know about home remedies yet, you'll probably get out some books on the subject. You may pull a book of children's symptoms off your shelf so you'll know what signs to look out for, or you may call an experienced mother or health care practitioner for more information. This is part of Step 1, "Gather information." As part of this step, you may choose to consult the section of this book on the physical exam and compare your findings with the pediatric symptoms book to make an educated guess about what is going on.

By now you may have prevented the cold from becoming too distressing, and the child is getting the extra nourishment she needs to gain full well-being. But let's just say that she wakes up in the night coughing deeply and harshly. You may decide to give her some chamomile tea (Step 3) or some herbal cough syrup and turn on a humidifier (Step 2). You prop up her pillows and stroke her head as she falls back to sleep (Steps 2 and 3). The next morning you continue to modify her diet with simple foods and provide the appropriate herbal remedies. This is applying Step 3. After a few days of treatment, rest, and loving, she is regaining her health.

But let's go a bit farther—just for those of you who really wonder about home health care. After about three days, your child's cough is not sounding any better. In fact, it is starting to sound deep and her fever is getting higher. You are starting to feel concerned and are unsure of what to do next for your child. Now you are at a crossroads. You may choose to continue your observation but under a time limit (Step1, "Gather information") and work with stronger herbal remedies (Step 4), you may choose to consult with someone (Step 2) more experienced with herbs and home health care than you, or you may feel that it is time for your child to see a physician. If you choose to go to a physician, you may receive a diagnosis that leaves you feeling comfortable about your child's situation and then decide to continue with the home remedies, or you may decide that medication is the best route (Step 5). Perhaps your doctor tells you that your child really seems to have pneumonia, but only a chest x-ray will give you a definitive diagnosis. You decide that you should know whether this is going on and opt for the x-ray. This is applying Step 6.

First and foremost, remember that you have to do what you feel you can live with and what is best for the child. Being stuck on the idea of home health care when a child needs to see a physician is no wiser than giving medication unnecessarily. Just make your choices from a place of clarity. All the choices described above are consistent with the Six Steps of Healing. As you come through each new situation, you will gain greater confidence. If you seek to make decisions not based solely on fear, greater numbers of possibilities will become apparent to you.

When you are using the Six Steps, circumstances may require that you go from Step 1 to Step 6 in a matter of seconds—for example, if your child sustains a severe injury. Whatever step you have gone to, if the situation is improving you can always go back to an earlier step. You can skip around or use a couple of steps at the same time.

❖ WHEN TO SEEK MEDICAL HELP ❖

Modern Western medicine is not inherently "bad." The main problem with conventional medicine is its overuse of medications and harmful procedures. But in cases of severe trauma and severe and worsening infections or diseases, it is at its best. Unfortunately, a family will occasionally become so reactive to what is perceived as "bad medicine" practiced by conventionally trained doctors that they will refuse medical care at all costs. You could say they are "throwing out the baby with the bathwater."

As parents, we have the great responsibility of deciding how to respond to our children's illnesses and accidents. We need to make the right decision, and that means putting aside our own distress. Remaining calm and clear minded when a child is ill is very challenging. We are inextricably bound to our children, and their health and survival is what we build many dreams upon. Remember that panicking will not change the situation. Instead, it interferes with your ability to choose the most sensible approach and creates unnecessary fear and anxiety in the child.

WHEN TO SEEK MEDICAL CARE

If your child is severely ill—hemorrhaging, unconscious, or displaying symptoms of a serious illness—seek *immediate emergency medical care*. If your treatment for a mild condition is not helping and the condition persists or worsens, quickly seek medical help or more experienced natural health care. Some conditions, like meningitis, appendicitis, bacterial pneumonia, and blood poisoning, can progress rapidly. Familiarize yourself with the symptoms of these illnesses in this book or a book on pediatric symptoms such as *A Parent's Guide to Childhood Symptoms*, by Dr. Richard Martin (see "Further Reading"). Some of these symptoms include fever with stiff neck, severe abdominal pain, red streaks emanating from a wound, and unremitting fever or cough accompanied by severe chest pain.

Remain calm and attentive, and you will be able to make the most appropriate choices.

Should your child require emergency care, stay close to him. Your presence will be very comforting. Hospitals may tell you that it is their policy not to allow parents into examination or treatment rooms. In fact, this may be their policy, but policies are different than laws. No law would support this policy. *Insist* on remaining with and comforting your child (and breast-feeding a young one).

Chapter 4

❖

Herbal Primer

The chapter is designed to provide readers with basic knowledge of the principles of herbalism and how to apply herbs for use in healing. It includes information that enables you to confidently interpret the general effects of herbal formulas, as well as how to obtain and prepare herbs for making your own herbal remedies.

❖ A Glossary of Herbal Properties ❖

The language in this book has been deliberately kept simple so that readers do not have to repeatedly refer to definitions. One of the ways the medical establishment maintains a "secret society" is through the use of complicated terms. We can demystify health care by making knowledge accessible to everyone. The following glossary of herbal properties is intended to help you understand the therapeutic action of herbs—that is, what they do in your body. The herbs listed after each definition are often used for maintaining and restoring children's health.

Alteratives: Create healthy changes in the blood; "blood purifiers." Tend to be cooling to the system in general. Include red clover blossoms, dandelion root, echinacea, plantain, chickweed, and burdock root.

Analgesics: Relieve pain. Include catnip, chamomile flowers, valerian root, skullcap, and lobelia.

Antiasthmatics: Help ease the symptoms of asthma. May relax the lungs, dilate the bronchioles, and help eliminate mucus. (Herbs specific to the lungs are known as "Pectorals.") Include comfrey, coltsfoot, mullein, lobelia, and wild cherry bark.

Antibiotics: Help stop the growth of or kill bacteria, viruses, or amoebas. Include echinacea, thyme, garlic, myrrh, chaparral, and goldenseal root.

Antihelmintics: Kill worms. (*See* Parasiticides and Vermifuges.)

Antipyretics: Also called "febrifuges." *Anti* means "against"; *pyre* means "fire." Reduce fever and cool the blood. Include chickweed, elder, echinacea, mints, honeysuckle, alfalfa, and seaweeds.

Antispasmodics: Prevent and relax muscle spasms. Include black cohosh, skullcap, lobelia, chamomile, valerian, hops, and passion flower.

Astringents: Tone and tighten tissue: tend to be drying as well. Use for treatment of diarrhea, skin problems, discharges, and hemorrhages. Include red raspberry leaf, blackberry root, witch hazel, calendula, myrrh, bayberry bark, white oak bark, and yellow dock root.

Carminatives: Relieve gas and griping (cramps in the bowels). Include anise, caraway, fennel, dill, ginger, peppermint, catnip, and chamomile.

Demulcents: Are soothing and relieve inflammation. Have a thick, slippery quality after steeping in hot water. Usually used internally for irritated tissue as in coughs or in the passage of kidney stones. Can be used externally as pastes to soothe dry or irritated skin. May be used to relieve constipation and to soothe urinary tract infections. Include marshmallow root, comfrey root, licorice root, slippery elm bark, burdock, chickweed, and flax seeds.

Diaphoretics: Make you sweat; drink them hot. Especially useful for fevers, influenza, and colds. Include lemon balm, ginger root, elder flowers, catnip, yarrow, peppermint, and sage.

Diuretics: Increase urination; help to treat urinary tract infections, inflammations occurring below the waist, skin problems, and kidney stones. Include dandelion root, nettles, plantain, uva ursi, elder flowers, and burdock root. Taken at room temperature or cool (more effective) when used to promote urination.

Emetics: Promote vomiting and thereby empty the stomach, usually only when taken in large quantities. Include lobelia, bayberry bark, and ipecacuanha. Traditionally used for croup or asthma by early American herbalists to promote the expulsion of mucus and also for accidental poisoning.

Emollients: Soothe, soften, and protect the skin. Include almond oil, olive oil and other vegetable oils, marshmallow root, comfrey root, slippery elm, and chickweed. (These herbs are also demulcents.)

Expectorants: Help clear mucus out of the lungs and throat. It is helpful to combine them with demulcents if a cough has caused irritation to the lungs and throat. Include anise seed, mullein, coltsfoot, wild cherry bark, sage, lobelia, and horehound.

Hemostatics: Stop hemorrhage. Include bayberry bark, shepherd's purse, witch hazel, white oak bark, yellow dock, and nettles.

Laxatives: Promote bowel movements. Range from mild (aperients) to very strong (cathartics). Cathartics are not generally used with kids. Gentle laxatives include licorice root, slippery elm, carob, yellow dock, dandelion, Irish moss, flax seeds, and psyllium seeds. A large enough quantity of nearly any warm beverage will act as a laxative.

Nervines: Effects range from calming and tonifying the nerves to strong sedation, depending on the strength of the preparation. Include chamomile, skullcap, hops, valerian, catnip, lemon balm, lavender, lady's slipper, passion flower, wood betony, and lobelia.

Parasiticides: Destroy parasites in the digestive tract and on the skin. Include garlic, black walnut, thyme, chaparral, and rue.

Stimulants: Enhance energy, stimulate circulation, and create warmth in the body. Often added in small amounts to other formulas to hasten the activity of herbs and to circulate herbs in the body. Include ginger root, cinnamon, anise seed, cayenne, garlic, bayberry bark, and angelica.

Tonics: Have a general strengthening effect on the whole person; also have specific effects on the organ systems they benefit. For example, there are heart tonics, nervous-system tonics, lung tonics, and liver tonics. Some tonic herbs are catnip (nerves), lemon balm (nerves), hawthorn berries (heart), dandelion root (liver), licorice root (general), and ginseng (vitality). Many more herbs belong to this category.

Vermifuges: Expel intestinal parasites. Include garlic, wormwood, fennel, chaparral, mugwort, and cayenne. Most are too strong tasting to be palatable for children and therefore present difficulty in usage.

Vulneraries: Help wounds heal. Include calendula, comfrey, aloe vera, slippery elm, and plantain.

❖ Herb Gathering ❖

Whether you plan to grow, gather from the wild, or purchase the herbs you use in your preparations and remedies, you are certain to find the process of making your own medicines fun and rewarding. In the long run, putting up a batch of herbal salve or earache oil that will last two years is less costly than purchasing expensive ointments and prescriptions for antibiotics. Although you may still need to buy a drugstore concoction on occasion, I think you will find yourself able to rely more and more on your home remedies. This is quite empowering. The greatest advantage is that kids gain a lot of knowledge when you let them assist in the preparations. Botany, environmental science, chemistry, cooking, and mathematics, to name a few topics, can be conveyed to your kids as you identify, harvest, weigh, mix, and cook your herbs. And the best part is that it's really fun!

From the Wild

Whenever possible, use herbs harvested from the wild in the area where you live. An uncultivated plant has more vitality than a cultivated one, just as wild animals retain more of their natural qualities than those living in zoos. Instruction in plant identification and harvesting is beyond the scope of this handbook, but I encourage you to learn to identify a few local medicinals to enhance your connection with the plant world.

If you are going to use local wild plants, be make *absolutely certain* that your plant identification is accurate. Mistakes can be fatal. Refer to "Further Reading" for a listing of field guides, and seek the advice of botanists at local nature centers. Never pick plants that grow near roads, under power lines, or in any other areas treated with or exposed to fertilizers, pesticides, toxic wastes, or other chemicals. Choose healthy plants far from the road in clean, unpolluted areas. Don't pick all of the plants in one location. Leave enough growing to repopulate the area. Avoid endangered or rare plant species. Always offer your thanks to the plants, and ask for their blessing and assistance in healing.

In Your Garden

Herb cultivation is a very broad field, one in which I am by no means an expert. I do know, however, that the greatest joy I find in herbs is when I am sitting in a garden filled with healing plants. Many herbs are not only useful but also beautiful, particularly when they are in bloom. Then the bees and butterflies will flock to your garden, and you will feel a new and profound connection to the plant world.

When you grow your own herbs, you develop a greater understanding of them. You see how they change through the seasons, what conditions cause them to thrive, and you learn to recognize their scent and appearance.

The initial investment in seeds or starter plants varies depending on how much you want to grow. A small garden well cared for can provide you with enough herbs to make small amounts of a few remedies. A large garden could potentially provide you with all of the herbs you could want and some to spare for friends or even for sale. Many herbs are prolific, so even a small plant, tended well, will yield a plentiful harvest over time. Perennials return year after year, so if your budget is limited, go with these instead of annuals, which die after the first year and may not always reseed. Not all herbs grow in every climate or location, so you need to consult books and local gardening stores to determine exactly what can be raised where you live. Books by the Rodale Press tend to be informative and interesting and are usually available at garden shops.

Purchasing Herbs

If you are buying dried herbs in the loose, bulk form from a health-food store, a mail-order catalog, or another source, it is preferable to obtain organic, wild-crafted plants or at least organically cultivated plants. Preparations such as capsules and tinctures should likewise be prepared from organic herbs. Many inorganic herbs are fumigated with fungicides and insecticides during storage, and some are even irradiated. Check your sources. All herbs and herb products should have a fresh smell, and their colors should resemble those of the fresh plants. Herb freshness will affect the potency and therefore the effectiveness of your treatments. A moldy odor indicates that the herbs are not fresh. Look closely for insects; one infested batch of herbs can let tons of bugs loose in your home. They can then infest other herbs in your pantry as well as get into your foods.

❖ HERBAL PREPARATIONS ❖

Seeing different herbs turn water, alcohol, and oils into lovely shades of gold, red, orange, green, and brown is nothing short of magic. Children will more readily take a remedy that looks more like a magical potion than a medicine, especially if they had a hand in preparing it. And for parents, preparing one's own remedies adds a special potency to the medicines: that of love and care.

Only common supplies are required for making everything from teas to salves in your kitchen: glass jars of varying sizes with lids, glass or stainless-steel pots, a sharp knife, a small funnel, a mesh strainer, a vegetable grater, measuring spoons, and a cutting board. Water, vegetable oil, vodka, and beeswax complete the list once you have the herbs you need.

Some preparations cannot be made easily at home. These include essential oils, which require special equipment for extraction, and herbs that must be powdered finely with a special grinder. If you wish, try experimenting with a coffee grinder to see if you achieve a powder that you find satisfactory.

If you plan to use your own preparations as your primary medicines, you will want to look through this book and plan ahead. Tinctures take weeks to prepare, for example, so you will need to have these on hand since you do not have weeks to wait if your child needs a tincture today. Otherwise, you will need to purchase the herbs and preparations as the need for them arises. Keep in mind that most herbal preparations such as oils and tinctures will keep for up to a few years (oils must be kept refrigerated), so if you prepare small batches of medicines at a time, you will find that little gets wasted.

FORMS OF PREPARATION

There are many ways to extract the elements from plants to prepare herbal remedies. Different types of preparations are required for different situations. Water, alcohol, and oil are the most common bases used (*menstruum* is another word for a base or solvent). Some herbalists also use vinegar, but since it is not suitable for all herbs, I reserve it for steeping fresh culinary herbs.

WATER BASES

The Earth, plants, and our bodies are primarily made of water, so our bodies accept water-based solutions easily. These include teas, infusions, decoctions, and syrups. Infusions and decoctions are used for baths, washes, and compresses as well as internal use.

Tea is the most basic herbal preparation. To make a tea, steep 1 teaspoon to 1 tablespoon of a dried herb in 1 cup boiling water for up to twenty minutes. Herbs with a lot of volatile oil content are easily extracted this way and so should be covered during steeping to prevent loss of their oils. Peppermint, catnip, lemon balm, chamomile, fresh ginger, lavender, and seeds such as fennel and anise are in this category.

Infusions are medicinal-strength teas. More herb material is steeped longer in slightly more water than is usual for a tea. The result is a darker, stronger-tasting, more potent brew. Pint- and quart-size canning (Mason) jars are the best vessels in which to make infusions.

To make an infusion, you usually steep 1 ounce of chopped, dried herb or 2 ounces of chopped, fresh herb in either a quart or pint jar filled with boiling water for anywhere from a half hour to eight hours. The amount of water in relation to plant material depends upon the strength desired for the remedy. The length of steeping time likewise corresponds to the intended strength of the remedy and upon the part of the plant being used. The general recommendations are as follows:

Roots: Use 1 ounce dried root to 1 pint of boiling water; steep for eight hours.

Bark: Prepare as for roots.

Leaves: In general, when preparing delicate leaves or those rich in essential oils, use 1 ounce of dried leaves or 2 ounces of fresh leaves to 1 quart of water and steep for one to two hours. Thick leaves (such as uva ursi) require steeping for up to six hours. Leaves used for nutritional purposes (such as nettles) should be steeped for up to eight hours.

Flowers: As these are delicate, steep 1 ounce of dried flowers in 1 quart of boiling water for a maximum of one hour.

Seeds: In general, you first gently crush the seeds with a mortar and pestle and then steep them for up to a half hour. Usually a 1/4 to 1/2 ounce of seeds per pint of water is sufficient.

Generally, dosage of an infusion ranges from 1/4 to 1 cup, two to four times daily. Sometimes an infusion is sipped throughout the day.

Decoctions are concentrated infusions. This makes for a strong brew that is taken in smaller dosages. A decoction is an excellent way to give herbs to children who otherwise might not tolerate large amounts of a strong-tasting preparation. The method is especially suited for nutrient roots such as yellow dock and dandelion because the child can get concentrated doses of minerals without having to drink cupfuls of beverage. Leaves, flowers, and seeds are rarely decocted as their constituents can be damaged by boiling.

To prepare a decoction, make an infusion and steep it for up to eight hours. Strain the liquid into a saucepan (discarding the used plant material), and gently simmer until it is reduced to one-quarter to one-half of the original amount. Take care not to boil away all of the liquid. It takes approximately an hour to reduce a pint of liquid by one-half (down to a cup). Pour into a glass jar, let cool to room temperature, and then refrigerate.

When unsweetened, decoctions last in the refrigerator for up to three days. Two tablespoons of honey per 1/2 cup of liquid or about 2 tablespoons of brandy per cup of liquid can extend the life of a decoction for up to three months when kept refrigerated.

Dosage is usually 1 teaspoon to 1 tablespoon, two to four times daily.

Syrups are easy to make from a decoction. Syrups have two main advantages over decoctions: Children will more readily take a small amount of a sweet-flavored medicine than any amount of an unpalatable one, and the large amount of sweetener in the syrup preserves the preparation, which helps it keep in the refrigerator for longer than even a sweetened decoction. Simply sweeten your decoction by adding an equal amount (by weight) of sweetener. One cup of a decoction is 8 ounces, so a decoction of this amount would require 8 ounces of sweetener. I use 1/4 to 1/2 cup of honey per cup of liquid and find this adequate; honey is considered to be twice as sweet as sugar. Add the sweetener to your hot decoction, bring to the boiling point while stirring, and then immediately pour into clean jars. Cool to room temperature, label, and refrigerate. Dosage is similar to a decoction but of course will vary from herb to herb.

Herbal baths are a rejuvenating ritual and are useful for all sorts of complaints: sore muscles, injured skin, exhaustion, irritability, congestion, and fever, to name a few. When using baths with children, be very careful to avoid burns from overly hot water.

A *foot bath* is given in a basin of water wide enough for the feet and deep enough to reach at least above the ankles. Add a quart of herbal infusion to enough hot water to fill the basin.

A *sitz bath* requires a quart of decoction or a couple of quarts of infusion placed in a shallow tub with enough water to reach hip level.

A *full bath* can be made two ways. One is to fill a cotton cloth or sock with at least an ounce of herbs and fasten the closed cloth to the faucet so bathwater runs through it while the tub is filling. Squeeze the sack now and then to wring out the "tea." This will make a mild but pleasant herbal bath. The second method is to prepare a couple of quarts of herbal infusion or decoction and then strain these into the tub of water.

If you keep the door to the bathroom closed, the aroma of the herbs and any volatile oils will fill the air, adding to the relaxing effect of the bath. Herb baths are a nourishing gift that children especially appreciate. Floating herb flowers on the water makes for a fun bath, but use a drain screen to keep the plant material from clogging your drain.

Steam baths can be used therapeutically for upper respiratory congestion and fevers. Saunas and sweat lodges are similarly used in many parts of the world. Following is a simplified version for your home. Children should always be accompanied by an adult in a steam bath and should be allowed to leave at any point when they have had enough. Hot water and steam can result in serious burns, so take extra precautions.

Fill a pot with a few quarts of water and bring it to a boil. Remove the pot from the stove and add a handful of herbs rich in volatile oils (mint, sage, and thyme work well) or up to 3 drops of essential oil (any of the above or eucalyptus). Cover immediately. Gather a couple of chairs, a large warm blanket (preferably wool), and your covered pot of hot water. Seat yourselves and place the covered pot near your feet. Being careful not to touch the pot, make a tent over yourself and your child with the blanket. When you are fully in, open the pot and breathe in the steam. When you have had enough, quickly dress and bundle up in bed.

Poultices and compresses are ways of applying herbs externally to specific areas of the body. You can quickly make a poultice by mashing, bruising, or even chewing fresh herbs into a pulpy mass and applying it to the affected area. You can also make one by mashing fresh or dried herbs (dried herbs will need to be moistened with warm water first), and spreading the material on a thin cotton cloth, which is then applied to the area. A hot-water bottle can be placed over the herbs or cloth to retain the warmth. Poultices are used for stings, bites, localized infections, wounds, boils, abscesses, swellings, and tumors.

To make a compress, soak a cloth in a hot infusion or decoction, wring out the excess liquid, and apply the cloth to the area. Replace the compress when it cools. As with a poultice, a hot-water bottle placed over the preparation retains heat.

Washes are just what they sound like: You wash the area with an infusion or decoction. For example, you may want to use an eyewash for conjunctivitis or a wash for a skin infection such as ringworm. Washes are an effective and simple external remedy.

ALCOHOL BASES

Alcohol is used for making tinctures, concentrated alcohol extracts of herbs. It is a valuable menstruum because certain plant substances can only be extracted by alcohol. Tinctures are concentrated, quick acting, and convenient (they can easily be transported in a small bottle), and they have a shelf life of many years. Because they are so concentrated, only a few drops are needed, making them particularly useful for children and for serious conditions when a higher dosage of herbs is required. Tinctures are also convenient for working parents who can't easily prepare infusions or decoctions every day. They are not, however, used when the nutritional aspects of herbs are being sought. For this one should use teas, infusions, decoctions, and syrups.

The amount of alcohol ingested by a child taking tinctures is fairly insignificant. If you are concerned about this, simply evaporate the alcohol by adding the dose of tincture to be taken to 1/4 cup of hot water and let it sit exposed to the air for a few minutes. Many tinctures can now be purchased in a glycerine base, which, in addition to containing no alcohol, lends a slightly sweet taste.

Making tinctures at home is fun and much less expensive than buying them. Tinctures made with fresh plant material are superior to those made from dried herbs. Whenever possible, obtain fresh herbs for your homemade tinctures or purchase tinctures made from fresh herbs. The best alcohol to use is 100-proof vodka, which is 50 percent alcohol and 50 percent water. Grain alcohol (almost 200 proof) or brandy can also be used. Brandy is nice for use in tinctures that will be given to very young kids because it is sweet and mildly warming, and it lacks a sharp alcohol taste.

Making tinctures: If you have gathered the herbs yourself, clean them by picking out damaged parts and brushing dirt off roots. Do not wash aboveground plant parts. Roots, stems, and bark need to be chopped. Place about 2 ounces of plant material in a pint jar. Fill the jar to the top with alcohol to lessen the possibility of spoilage. Cap the jar tightly and label it with the name of the herb, alcohol content, and the date. Store where it won't be exposed to direct sunlight, and give it a gentle shake every few days. If you see the liquid level going down, top off the jar with some more alcohol.

Some folks let their tinctures "work" for only two weeks. I prefer to let mine tincture for six weeks, starting at the new moon and ending at the full moon six weeks later. The moon, which exerts ongoing effects on the Earth, including the level of oceans and the growth of plants, as well as our own internal regulatory mechanisms, such as hormones or menstrual flow in women, is also said to have an effect on the making of herbal tinctures. By beginning tinctures at the new moon we allow the full drawing effect of the moon to influence our preparations, drawing the properties of the herbs into the medium into which we are extracting the plant substances.

After six weeks, thoroughly strain the alcohol tincture from the plant material. This usually requires some vigorous wringing of the herbs in cheesecloth or cotton muslin to extract as much of the liquid as possible. Pour the tincture into well-labeled glass jars or tincture bottles (the jars need not be filled to the top) and store in a cool, dark place such as a pantry or the refrigerator.

Dosage of a tincture depends on the herbs used, the condition being treated, and the person's age and weight. Usually between 5 and 25 drops are taken four times a day. Store tinctures out of reach of children, an overdose could make them sick. Tinctures remain good for a minimum of two to three years.

Making liniments: These are tinctures prepared for external use in the treatment of muscle and ligament trauma. They tend to contain herbs that act as local stimulants (for example, angelica, cinnamon, wintergreen, cayenne, calendula) in order to bring deep warmth to the affected area and disperse blood congestion to reduce bruising. The alcohol (use vodka or other 100-proof alcohol) makes them quick absorbing and penetrating. Prepare as for tinctures, or add essential oils to an alcohol base. Apply by rubbing enough into the skin to cover the sore or bruised area. Do not use on broken skin.

OIL BASES

Herbal oils, salves, and ointments can be made at home. Essential oils are highly concentrated plant extracts that cannot easily be made at home and are rarely used internally because their strength can be fatal. I have occasionally suggested the use of essential oils in this book as external remedies, and caution you to store them out of the reach of children.

Herbal oils, sometimes called "medicated oils," are vegetable oils in which herbs have been infused. They are different from essential oils, which are derived by extracting large volumes of concentrated, active chemical ingredients from plants. Herbal oils are used in the treatment of sore muscles, sprains, aches, infections, and irritated skin, as well as for massage. Many herbal oils mentioned in this book can be used on broken skin, although arnica oil cannot.

To make an herbal oil, loosely fill a clean and totally dry jar with dry herbs. Now fill the jar to the brim with oil. Almond, olive, and sesame oils are the most commonly used, but any vegetable oil is acceptable. Store at room temperature in partial sunlight for one to four weeks. Some herbs, such as garlic and rosemary, will keep well in oil for the longer time span, while other herbs, particularly the more delicate plants and plant parts such as chickweed and rose petals, will begin to spoil after a week. Hot weather will cause the plants and oil to spoil more quickly, whereas plants extracted in a cool environment will keep longer before you must decant them. Direct light and heat should be avoided. Infuse and store on a surface that will not be damaged by any oil seepage that may occur. At the end of the given time period, strain well and store in a cool, dark place or refrigerate. Oils will keep for up to a year or more, and are considered good as long as they do not turn rancid. A rancid oil has a peculiar smell that is distinctly different from either the smell of the fresh oil or the plant being steeped. If you suspect that your oil has turned, discard it and begin anew.

Salves are used for healing skin injuries: wounds, burns, stings, rashes, sores, and the like. Salve can be made a few different ways, all of which are effective. This first method is preferable because it requires less cooking time than the others, thereby retaining more of the subtle properties of the herbs. Prepare an herbal oil from your desired ingredients; then pour it into a small pot. To this add grated beeswax, 1 tablespoon per ounce of oil. Heat over a low flame until the wax is melted. To test for readiness, put a small amount onto a teaspoon and place it in the refrigerator. After a minute it will harden to its finished consistency. Salve should be firm and solid but not so hard that it won't melt into your skin. If the consistency is correct, pour your salve into small jars, cool to room temperature, cover, and store. If the salve is too soft, add more beeswax; if it is too hard, add more oil.

A second method is to place about an ounce of herbs and 1/3 cup of oil in a small pot. Simmer for two hours on a *very low* flame with the pot covered. Add a bit of oil if necessary, and watch carefully to avoid scorching. After cooking, strain the herbs well through a cotton cloth or cheesecloth, squeezing as much of the oil as possible out of the plant material. You may need to let the oil cool before this can be done. Clean the pot and dry it (discarding the used plant material); then pour the oil back in, adding a couple tablespoons of grated beeswax. Melt this over a low flame, stirring constantly. Check for readiness as in the first method; then bottle and store.

Another method requires less watching. Mix 4 ounces of oil, 1 ounce of herb, and 1/2 ounce of beeswax in an ovenproof pot. Cover the pot and bake the mixture for about three hours at 250 degrees Fahrenheit. Strain through cheesecloth, bottle, and store.

Salves will keep for a couple of years if stored in the refrigerator, about a year if not. To extend the life of your salve to the full two years, you can add 1 teaspoon of vitamin E oil or 1 to 2 tablespoons of an herbal tincture per 4 ounces of salve (while still warm, before bottling). Any herbal tincture will work, as it is the alcohol that helps preserve it, but to increase the healing qualities of your salve, use a tincture with either skin healing or antimicrobial properties. Both echinacea and calendula tinctures make good choices for use in herbal salves.

Ointments are prepared exactly like salves, but less beeswax is used in order to obtain a softer product. Cutting the amount of beeswax by half should yield a desirable consistency.

When you experiment in your kitchen pharmacy, above all enjoy yourself. Of course it's best not to be wasteful, but don't worry if you make a mistake and have to discard something. Compost piles are very forgiving. Try to be patient and learn from your mistakes. Be persistent; the rewards are worth it!

❖ DOSAGES ❖

Dosage of any herbal remedy depends upon three factors: (1) the age and weight of the person, (2) the strength of the preparation, and (3) the severity of the condition being treated. Most herbals geared toward adults give dosages for a 125- to 150-pound adult. When using general herbals for kids, reduce the stated dosage proportionally.

In this book, recommended dosages are given in a range geared toward children of average weight and size, between the ages of two and twelve years. In general, the younger and slimmer the child, the lower the dosage. The dosages given in Part II, "Newborn and Baby Care," are specifically for children under two years of age.

If a remedy seems ineffective, you may need to increase the dosage slightly. However, don't give more just to achieve faster results—herbal medications don't work on a "more is better" principle. Likewise, if you notice any undesirable effects from an herbal medication, decrease the dosage or discontinue that preparation.

❖ An Herbal Medicine Chest ❖

Using herbs as your primary medicines requires forethought. Although most herbs are available at health-food stores and can be purchased during business hours, illnesses do not always arise when it is convenient; nor can you always take a sick child shopping. While you can usually find a twenty-four-hour pharmacy to purchase needed drugs (and some even deliver!), that is not the case with herbal medicines. The herbs listed below are useful to have on hand. Keeping a supply of herbs and premade remedies also encourages you to use them regularly for nutrition and prevention of illness. It is helpful to have dried herbs in bulk easily accessible and certain remedies premade.

Two to 4 ounces of each (dried) herb you choose to keep on hand and a few tinctures will probably suffice. Store herbs either in amber-colored bottles or in a spot out of direct sunlight. Keep them away from heat as well. Storing bulk herbs in the freezer can reduce insect infestation, which can occur over time.

You do not have to get every item on the following list, but choose an assortment that will cover a broad range of uses. This is not an exhaustive list of all the plant remedies found in this book although they are the most repeatedly used. For a thorough home health kit, you will also want to have an herbal first-aid kit on hand; see Appendix II.

In the list, each herb's common name is followed by its Latin, or horticultural, name. When purchasing an herb, check its Latin name because many different herbs can have the same common name.

Dried herbs are frequently used, primarily because fresh plants may not be available year-round, if at all. Fresh herbs can be substituted for dry herbs, as can tinctures. Throughout this book, if a certain form of an herb or preparation is better than another—for example, use of a tincture over a tea, or a fresh herb over a dried herb—that preference is so noted.

Anise seed (*Pimpinella anisum*): Generally considered a culinary herb, anise is also a useful medicine that prevents and relieves intestinal gas and is helpful in relieving coughs. Its pleasant taste makes it palatable to even very young children.

Burdock root (*Arctium lappa*): Burdock is both tonifying and purifying for the blood. It is useful both internally and externally for infections and most skin problems. Burdock is a nourishing food with a pleasant, sweet taste; when purchased fresh, it may be prepared as a vegetable.

Calendula (*Calendula officinalis*): This healer from the marigold family is beautiful and remarkably effective for the treatment of internal and external injuries, irritations, and inflammations. It is an excellent antiseptic and soothing treatment for burns and cuts. It relieves the itch and sting of insect bites, and in the form of an oil it heals skin rashes.

Catnip (*Nepeta cataria*): An essential herb to keep stocked if you have small children, this plant in the mint family calms an irritable child, induces sweating to assist in a fever, and helps relieve indigestion and achiness.

Chamomile (*Chamaemelum nobile* or *Matricaria recutita*): I think chamomile is really an angel in plant form. It reduces stress, anxiety, fear, pain, aches, and restlessness. Its pretty golden orange flowers make an excellent tea for bedtime, stomach troubles, inflammation, insomnia, and "flu-ishness." It can be used as a wash for irritated eyes or as a mouthwash for oral inflammations. Compresses are soothing for bruises and wounds. Nursing mothers will quickly befriend this calcium-rich herb, which has benefits both for themselves and their children.

Cinnamon (*Cinnamomum zeylanicum*): Cinnamon aids digestion, nausea, and vomiting. It lends warmth to the body and stops diarrhea. In liniments it eases sore muscles.

Comfrey (*Symphytum officinale*): Both the leaves and root of this hardy perennial are healing for those with diarrhea, broken bones, injured tissue, and coughs. Comfrey is nutritious and is said to be one of the few vegetable sources of Vitamin B_{12}.

Echinacea (*Echinacea angustifolia*): Known for its abilities as a blood purifier and antimicrobial, echinacea is a very important herb to use during infections and can also be used externally as a wash for wounds. Its cooling nature reduces inflammation, fever, and infection. It is also used to treat poisonous bites and stings. I use echinacea tincture made from fresh plants only unless I have fresh plants available for an infusion. Echinacea is most effective when used fresh and is a superb immune-system tonic. It can be used to prevent illness.

Elder Flowers (*Sambucus nigra*): These flowers of the versatile elder tree are noted for their effectiveness in assisting children and adults with high fevers. Combine it with peppermint in equal parts to avoid digestive upsets.

Garlic (*Allium sativum*): Garlic is a strong medicine-food known to be antimicrobial. That is, it is both antiviral and antibacterial. It is especially helpful in treating upper respiratory infections and earaches; it is also considered useful in eliminating intestinal parasites. In addition, garlic is a tonic and can help regulate both high and low blood pressure. Used as a regular part of a diet, it can boost the immune system. It is used raw or in tea, syrup, or oil. Keep both fresh garlic bulbs and garlic oil on hand.

Ginger (*Zingiber officinale*): Ginger root is probably my favorite adult remedy for fevers, colds, and chills. It stimulates the circulation, breaks up congestion, and brings out a good sweat. Ginger is used internally for both arthritis and muscle aches, and its juice has even been used to treat burns. It is an excellent remedy for stomach upset, nausea, and car sickness. Some children love the taste of ginger tea with honey; others find it too spicy.

Goldenseal (*Hydrastis canadensis*): I rarely use goldenseal right off because it is so strong that I consider it almost a drug—an antibiotic, to be precise. I have seen it clear up even serious dysentery. It is an important herb, and it is good to stock both the powder and tincture in case of persistent or serious infection.

Lemon Balm (*Melissa officinalis*): Lemon balm is a gentle and effective soother, nerve quieter, and fever assistant with a pleasant taste. This age-old remedy for ill children combines well with catnip and chamomile.

Licorice (*Glycyrrhiza glabra*): Sweet and soothing, licorice can be used to calm stomachs, reduce coughs, and balance the effects of strong herbs in formulas. Because it has a strong influence on the glandular system, it should not be used daily by children. It is an ingredient in the homemade cough syrup formula we keep in our medicine chest.

Lobelia (*Lobelia inflata*): Lobelia relaxes the system while it stimulates the lungs, making it especially useful for coughs and asthma. In high doses it can have toxic side effects, so carefully follow directions. Symptoms of too high a dose include stomach cramping and pain, nausea, vomiting, headache, or any unusual symptom that was not present before. If this occurs, just stop using it for a while, and if you use it again use a lower dose. I know of no lasting harmful side effects.

Marshmallow root (*Althea officinalis*): Marshmallow is a highly mucilaginous plant that aids in soothing coughs and other respiratory irritations, inflammations of the mouth and digestive tract, and urinary tract inflammations. It can also be used externally for inflammations.

Mullein (*Verbascum thapsus*): The velvety leaves of this plant are used in cough syrup; the oil of the leaves and flowers is a must for reducing the pain associated with earaches. Mullein oil is also useful for treating skin inflammations.

Nettles (*Urtica dioica*): Nettles strengthens the whole body and, being nutritious, is an excellent regular addition to our diets. It builds the blood and nourishes the kidneys and circulatory system.

Peppermint (*Mentha piperita*): Peppermint grows easily in gardens, even with poor soil. It makes a cool, light, and refreshing beverage; aids digestion; and soothes stomach aches. When combined with other herbs, such as elder blossoms, it makes a tea good for soothing a feverish child.

Red clover (*Trifolium pratense*): Red clover is a pleasant-tasting, blood-nourishing herb that can be used to treat skin conditions, coughs, and blood infections.

Red raspberry leaf (*Rubus idaeus*): Raspberry leaves are probably most known for their use during pregnancy, but they are equally useful in resolving diarrhea and sore throats because of their strong astringent properties. They are a nutritious tonic and can be used regularly.

Skullcap (*Scutellaria laterifolia*): A safe and effective nerve tonic, skullcap combines well with many of the other nervines. Tincture is an excellent form for giving this herb to children. It is gentle and can be used regularly in small doses.

Slippery elm bark (*Ulmus fulva*): This herb is almost foolproof for eliminating constipation in babies. Slippery elm is mucilaginous, meaning it gets gelatinous when mixed with a liquid. It is an important ingredient in many cough formulas and, when combined with powdered ginger and licorice, makes delicious lozenges. Slippery elm can be used externally for chafed skin and diaper rash. It tastes much like maple syrup and can be sprinkled in porridge or blended into "smoothies" and puddings to increase their nutritional value.

Thyme (*Thymus vulgaris*): Thyme has strong antimicrobial properties and can be used for cleansing infected wounds, for eliminating respiratory and digestive infections, and for relieving diarrhea. A hair wash made from the oil eliminates head lice.

Valerian (*Valeriana officinalis*): Valerian will relieve cramps, tension, and toothaches (apply the tincture directly to the tooth). A small amount rubbed into the gums of a teething baby brings relief. This herb is especially useful for children who tend to get "hyper."

Wild cherry bark (*Prunus serotina*): A common ingredient in cough syrup, wild cherry bark relaxes the muscles of the chest, easing bronchitis, and irritable coughs. It brings relief even in cases of whooping cough. Overdose is possible; use in small amounts as part of a formula.

Other items: You may find the following items mentioned for a specific condition in this book, and therefore may want to have these on hand:

- Hydrogen peroxide
- Bach Rescue Remedy
- Pure honey: Antiseptic and delicious, but because of botulinus spore it is unsafe for children under fifteen months of age.
- Herbal salve
- Lemons: Cooling, they add flavor and nutrition to herb tea and can be combined with honey as a simple remedy for sore throats.
- Activated charcoal (carbon derived from organic material and

treated with oxygen, steam, and high temperature to increase the internal and external surface areas and pores, giving it great adsorptive properties): Excellent for providing relief from severe indigestion and migraine-type headaches. It is an antidote in some types of accidental poisonings.

- Ipecac: Available at any pharmacy, this syrup causes vomiting and is used for accidental poisoning. (Always contact your local poison-control center before inducing vomiting.)
- Vitamin C (tablets or crystals): Helps prevent or reduce infection in many cases.
- Essential oils (such as thyme, eucalyptus, and peppermint): All make nice additions to baths as well as steams for chest congestion.
- Green clay: Available at most natural foods stores, green clay makes an excellent poultice for drawing out abscesses and stings.
- Apple cider vinegar: This old home remedy is an internal and external antiseptic and is used to treat fungal infections such as thrush and ringworm. It is very rich in B vitamins.
- Sea salt: Keep about 2 cups on hand. Use in mouth rinses for toothache and gum inflammation and in a salt pack for vomiting and diarrhea.
- Homeopathic remedies: Arnica 30x is invaluable for treating muscle aches, bruises, and sprains. It can be given after any trauma. *Note:* The notation "30x" is a unit of measurement in homeopathic medicine referring to the strength of the preparation. The number indicates how many times the original substance was diluted. The *x* following the number means that it was diluted in decimal potencies, 1 part medicine to 9 parts water, alcohol, or powdered milk sugar (lactose). Common dilutions are 3, 6, 30, 200, 1,000, and even higher. Homeopathic remedies may also be diluted in centesimal amounts (that is, 1 part medicine to 99 parts of another substance), in which case a *c* will appear after the number. The greater the number of dilutions, the less of the original substance contained in the final product, and the *stronger* the remedy. Homeopathic medications are shaken vigorously between dilutions, which is considered to *potentize* the medicine (lend it its active potential).
- In addition, many of the ingredients in the Herbal First-Aid Kit (see Appendix II) are helpful to have in the home and should be available should an accident occur. For example, Antispasmodic Tincture (available through Herb Pharm) is a sedating tincture used for fright and severe injury causing pain. Children's Compound

(also from Herb Pharm) is useful for calming fussy children as well as reducing fevers and associated discomfort. Tiger Balm, an analgesic salve, brings heat to the area where it is applied, reducing the discomfort of sprains and muscle aches, and, like a mentholated balm, improves breathing when applied sparingly to the chest for chest congestion. Avoid contact with broken skin, mucous membranes, and eyes, as it burns.

PART II

NEWBORN
AND
BABY CARE

Chapter 5

❖

Conception through Birth: Laying the Foundation

While extensive discussion of fetal development and childbirth is beyond the scope of this book, a book on children's health would be incomplete without at least a brief treatment of these topics. Just as you would not build a beautiful home on a weak foundation, a child's wellbeing depends to a large extent on the prenatal and early postnatal health care he or she receives. This chapter provides insight into the ways in which women can use natural remedies and practical information to maintain or improve their health during pregnancy, prepare for birth, and care for themselves and their newborns in the days and months after birth. If you are already pregnant and feel you haven't been as conscientious about your health as you would like, don't despair—foundations can always be reinforced, and babies are very forgiving!

Men who are participating in the care of their pregnant partners and their babies will want to read this chapter as well. Now more than ever, your partner needs excellent nutrition, rest, and exercise, not to mention your support and assistance to help her take care of herself, which will be especially necessary if you already have younger children to care for. Like most men, you'll probably discover that your participation in the process of pregnancy and birth will enrich your experience as a man, as a father, and as a couple.

A child's body, quite literally, is begun at the time of conception, the product of mother and father. Ideally, *both* parents will work toward excellent health in the months prior to conception by eating a diet of natural foods, getting into good physical shape, and avoiding harmful substances such as drugs and environmental contaminants. The emotional, mental, and psychic state of the parents adds to the health of the developing child. Life definitely begins before birth.

For more extensive information on the overall aspects of health during pregnancy and on preparing for childbirth, refer to "Further Reading" and contact Cascade Health Care Products (see "Resources") for a book catalog.

❖ Eating Well During Pregnancy ❖

Food is a big issue for many women who strive to have bodies that meet American social standards of beauty. During pregnancy these standards are particularly dangerous to our physical and mental health and can interfere with proper nourishment. The most fundamental dietary "rule" during pregnancy is to eat mostly high-quality, whole foods: whole grains (eat a variety of whole grains including brown rice and millet, not just wheat), lots of fresh vegetables, fruit, good-quality protein (beans, seeds, and organic meats, for example), and plenty of water and herbal teas that support pregnancy. Eat whenever you feel hungry and don't skimp! Dairy foods are excellent in moderation, but drinking milk and eating large quantities of dairy foods daily can make for babies that are too big for a smooth vaginal birth. In addition, the many chemicals fed to dairy cows to increase their milk production may be less than healthy for you and your baby. Avoid the harmful chemical residues that are present both in and on produce by eating only organically grown fruits and vegetables.

I frequently work with women whose vegetable intake is extremely limited. Before and during pregnancy (even if you have to get used to the tastes and make an effort to prepare them), learn to eat a wide variety of veggies, especially dark, leafy greens such as collards, kale, broccoli and green lettuces such as romaine and green leaf, at least once (preferably twice) a day. Also, eat squashes, sweet potatoes, and lots of carrots regularly. You will derive a rich assortment of nutrients from these foods (vitamins A and C, folic acid, calcium, and iron, to name a few), will have excellent digestion, and will be harmonizing your body with nature much more than if you rely on processed or quick foods. The effort you put into caring for yourself during pregnancy is a meditation for a healthy birth and baby.

You don't have to weigh yourself regularly. Weighing yourself does not tell you that you are eating well, only that you're gaining weight. Weight gain is a misleading indicator of good nutrition because one can certainly gain weight on nonnutritious foods. Weight gain is a very individual matter, depending to some degree on your prepregnancy weight. Twenty to 40 pounds is considered the ideal range for pregnancy weight increase, but women who start pregnancy at or under 100 pounds may gain more, and heavier women may gain less. The most important factor seems to be a steady weight increase on healthy foods. If you eat a high-quality diet, you are unlikely to gain more or less than the perfect amount for you and your baby. You will need a little extra padding as reserves for birth and breast-feeding, so try not to worry. On the other hand, gaining a huge amount and having a big baby is not more desirable than having a good-size baby who easily fits through your pelvis and birth canal.

This is a time when it is essential to listen closely to your body's messages. When you feel hungry, it is essential that you take the time to eat. During pregnancy, irritability, weepiness, restlessness, insomnia, dizziness, and fatigue are hunger messages. Frequently, eating a high protein snack such as yogurt, cheese and crackers, peanut butter on toast, or a piece of baked chicken will miraculously resolve your discomfort. Even if you have to eat in the middle of the night, do so. Your body is working twenty-four hours a day to meet your baby's needs.

❖ CONNECTING WITH THE BABY IN YOUR WOMB ❖

Though "unseen," a baby in the womb requires no less love or care than a newborn. Prenatal babies thrive on being talked to, massaged through the mother's belly, and being well fed, both literally and spiritually, by both parents. Taking the time to be intimate with your baby and your partner can strengthen your marital relationship as well.

Over the years, studies done by physicians and psychologists such as Thomas Verny, David Chamberlain, and the many members of the Pre- and Peri-Natal Psychology Association of North America (PPANA) have consistently demonstrated that babies are able to learn in the womb and that they remember many things from their prenatal experiences. For example, babies recognize music that their parents played regularly or stories they read repeatedly during the pregnancy. There have even been recorded incidents of parents teaching their children advanced math and other academic subjects during gestation and the children then showing remarkable proficiency in them in early childhood, often before other children of their own age were learning to read. Children have also been known to relay memories of incidents that happened while their mothers were pregnant with them, incidents the parents themselves had never mentioned to them. The downside of all of this is that external factors also negatively affect unborn babies. For example, unborn babies exposed to hard rock music are known to move violently in the womb. Babies born to parents who fight frequently may experience more health problems in the neonatal period; even more disturbing is their capacity to retain the memories of painful experiences and the profound influence these experiences may have throughout life. Dr. Stanislav Grof and others have recorded a tendency toward depression and suicidal thought in children whose mothers had attempted aborting them during pregnancy. It is through psychotherapeutic techniques with depressed and suicidal patients that these memories first surfaced and were later confirmed in correspondence with their mothers or other close relatives. If you are interested in learning more about perinatal psychology, read *The Holotropic Mind*, by Stanislav Grof; *The Secret Life of the Unborn Child*, by Thomas Verny; and *Babies Remember Birth: Extraordinary Discoveries About the Mind and Personality of Newborns*, by David Chamberlain.

What is most positive about this knowledge is that we can provide our children, to the best of our ability, with security, love, and a deep sense of being wanted before they are born. But you don't have to be super-vigilant: Having fears and doubts about becoming a parent is completely normal. Most mothers and fathers experience some amount of ambivalence at least once during pregnancy when they realize how much responsibility they have and how much of their freedom they will have to give up. Nor can we totally control our external environment. Yes, we can avoid heavy metal music and play soothing classical music or Native American flute music instead, but we cannot always prevent a relative from becoming ill or a car from breaking down. We don't have to go off to some idyllic retreat for the entirety of our pregnancies, but we can learn to communicate to our babies during the stressful times that, yes, we are going through stress (or doubt, sadness, grief, anger) but it is not the baby's fault, and we still love the baby. Both parents can express this verbally, through touching the mother's belly or even by taking a few minutes here and there throughout the day to relax and send good thoughts to the child. These simple gestures can go a long way toward creating an emotionally healthy place for the baby. The father can do his best to shield his pregnant partner from unnecessary upsets during the pregnancy, such as not discussing stories in the news that may upset her and avoiding arguments about trivial issues. A few books offering suggestions for prenatal communication with your baby include *Bonding Before Birth*, by Leni Schwartz; *The Child of Your Dreams,* by Laura Huxley and Piero Ferrucci; and *Cradle of Heaven*, by Murshida Vera.

❖ HERBAL ALLIES FOR PREGNANCY ❖

Many herbs can provide you with additional nutrients, improve the health and functioning of your organs, and tonify your body in preparation for birth. This section discusses some of the herbs commonly used with good results and no known harmful side effects by many midwives currently practicing in the United States and in Europe. In addition, many herbs can be used in the prevention and treatment of common pregnancy discomforts and problems. For information about these, refer to "Further Reading."

In general, herbs used for enhancing nutrient levels and for tonification are taken as infusions. Some herbal preparations may seem unpalatable during early pregnancy but are quite pleasant later on, so if you can't stomach them at first, try again at a later date. *Don't take herbs during your pregnancy unless you are absolutely certain they are safe. Herbs are powerful and can have harmful effects on you and your baby if they are not safe for pregnancy.*

A general dosage for herbal infusions during pregnancy is 1 to 4 cups daily. Up to a quart of nutritious brews can be taken each day, but even just 1 cup a day will be beneficial. For preparation instructions see "Herbal Preparations" in Chapter 4.

My favorite herb for pregnancy is nettles. It is an excellent blood and circulatory system tonic that also strengthens the urinary tract. It prevents anemia, varicosities, kidney and bladder infections, and glucosuria (sugar in the urine)—all important for a healthy pregnancy— and even hemorrhaging at the time of birth.

Pregnant women enjoy drinking Nourishment Tea; in fact, the whole family will probably like this beverage. You can drink it plain, sweetened, or jazzed up with lemon. The herbs are both nutritious and tonifying. The tea may be used freely throughout the pregnancy and into the post-partum to promote milk production.

The Nourishment Tea recipe uses dried herbs in the following amounts: 1 ounce red raspberry leaves, 1 ounce nettles, 1 ounce oat-straw, 1/2 ounce alfalfa, 1/2 ounce red clover blossoms, 1/2 ounce comfrey leaves, and 1/4 to 1/2 ounce peppermint leaves. Mix all of the herbs and store away from heat and sunlight in a glass bottle or plastic bag. Use a handful of the mixture per quart of boiling water and steep for one hour for maximum benefit. Steep for less time if you find the taste becomes too strong after a long steeping.

Another excellent herbal preparation for pregnancy is an iron tonic syrup containing dandelion root and yellow dock root (see "Anemia [Iron Deficiency]" in Chapter 9). Take 1 to 2 tablespoons daily for enhancing iron levels as well as iron absorption. This tonic will also promote healthy liver functioning and improve bowel movements in the event of constipation.

Dandelion is an excellent general health promoter that improves appetite, reduces skin complaints, and promotes general well-being during pregnancy. Both the root and leaves can be used; the greens are a wonderful vegetable.

During the last four weeks of pregnancy, women can use a late-pregnancy tonic to promote uterine strength, balance the hormones, and encourage uterine contractions to begin (though this formula will *not* induce labor). A beneficial formula (using dried herbs) is 1 ounce red raspberry leaves, 1/2 ounce squawvine, and 1/4 ounce each of cramp bark, wild yam, and blue cohosh. Prepare by infusing 2 tablespoons of the above mixture in 1 quart of boiling water for one hour. Strain and drink 1 cup a day. If the drink is unpalatable, mix into a cup of red raspberry leaf tea tinctures of the other four herbs (5 drops each).

❖ CHOOSING THE BIRTHPLACE ❖

Your choice of birthplace is a personal one and should be made with care, confidence, and independent thought. Those who will feel comfortable if medical resources are immediately available probably will have an easier time at a birthing center or hospital than at home. While births in a medical environment can't be as natural as at home, they still can be beautiful if the mother and father accept the challenges of labor and birth with confidence, determination, and enthusiasm. Fear in itself can lead the body down a road of complications, so the mother's sense of security is paramount.

During your pregnancy you can educate yourself about the pros and cons of various interventions and the ways they can affect your birth experience and your baby's health. Two excellent books are *Special Delivery*, by Rahima Baldwin, a well-known childbirth educator and founder of Informed Birth/Homebirth and Parenting; and *The Birth Book*, by William and Martha Sears, a doctor-and-nurse couple who have eight children. Both books advocate informed choice and are supportive of both home birth and noninterventional hospital birth.

I am a firm advocate of home birth for those who feel deeply comfortable with that choice. I have birthed all four of my children at home, and all the births have been joyous experiences in which I felt very powerful. The pregnancies were trouble-free with the exception of first-trimester nausea, and the births likewise went very smoothly. I have not had "painless" births, however; all were initiations into my inner strength. My mate and I chose home birth not out of hatred for hospitals or the medical profession but out of a desire to quietly and peacefully welcome our children into the world, much as they were conceived.

❖ DEALING WITH FEARS ❖

No matter where the birth will take place, the mother must face and overcome fears of birth and mothering during her pregnancy. The father needs to look at his fears of becoming a dad, of responsibility, and of birth. Because birth cannot truly be "planned" and carries inherent risks, there is a natural element of fear that arises. Yet birth happens most easily when you enjoy a sense of trust and can give up the physical resistance inherent in the act of trying to control events. An ability to be spontaneous and flexible (to "go with the flow") facilitates birth. In fact, some midwives say that the length of labor and the likelihood of a cesarean increase with the length of the birth plan, a list of do's and don'ts created by the birthing mother or couple for the caregivers regarding care of the mother and baby. This is because a birth plan is often based on the fear that one's desires for a birth are incongruent with those of one's caregivers or the birth environment. On some internal level you may still be harboring fears or expectations about the birth that will impede your ability to trust, open, and relax into your birthplace. Trust in and love for your body are essential. It is natural and normal for fears to arise. You are facing a great unknown. But you don't have to invite your fears to a tea party. Let them come if they must, but then let them go with affirmations of trust in yourself.

Learning to relax and tune in to your body are the first steps in identifying fears. This is because fear, being a primal response to a threat against survival, registers first in the body as a "fight-or-flight" response. Unresolved fears can cause you to maintain tension constantly to a greater or lesser degree, depending upon the intensity of the fear. A tight gut, a tight behind, fast breathing, spontaneous sweating, and a quick pulse or heartbeat when thinking about the upcoming experience of birth are all signs that you have unresolved anxieties. By identifying where in your body you are holding anxiety, you can begin to release the tension from both your mind and body. Techniques that can assist you in this work include visualization, meditation, massage, journal writing, and the support of an experienced guide or counselor. For further information and techniques, consult books such as *Birthing Normally*, by Gayle Peterson; *Pregnancy as Healing*, by Gayle Peterson and Lewis Mehl; *Pregnant Feelings*, by Rahima Baldwin and Terra Palmarini; and *Transformation Through Birth*, by Claudia Panuthos.

❖ LABOR AND BIRTH ❖

Labor and birth are profound, life-changing experiences. They cause us to draw upon resources within ourselves that we often don't even realize we have. It would require a book in itself to share in depth the many ways that women, couples, and families can prepare themselves and the many options available for relaxation, birth settings, and even positions in which women can labor and birth. A wealth of material has been published on these topics; see "Further Reading" for selections that may interest you.

Rather than viewing pregnancy and birth as life-affirming events, our society tends to regard them as diseases that require the monitoring and medical expertise of obstetricians. The pervasiveness of this view is reflected in the fact that less than 1 percent of the American population gives birth at home, and that midwives are illegal in most states. Women are encouraged to undergo numerous and regular tests throughout pregnancy and labor to verify whether things are proceeding according to what the American College of Obstetricians and Gynecologists (ACOG) has deemed as "normal." Most women born in this culture have internalized these views, which is unfortunate and unnecessary. It robs us of the chance to experience the beauty and power that is inherent in our bodies' ability to carry and birth our babies. In contrast, pregnancy and birth are considered normal processes in most European countries. Women receive prenatal care primarily from midwives, who then assist in home birthing. The countries with the highest rates of midwife-assisted births and home births also have the lowest rates of infant mortality and morbidity in the world.

The reasons for the negative beliefs about birth so rampant in our culture are not dissimilar to the history of herbalism and natural healing in the United States. Changing these negative beliefs begins with each of us, and it is important that we do so. In a very real way, our ability to regain trust in our capacity to give birth is related to our ability to trust in our children's capacity to maintain health without unnecessary monitoring and intervention.

Start by taking time every day during your pregnancy, even if just for a few minutes, to affirm your ability to give birth. Spending time in nature—watching the miracle and perfection of a flower opening, a plant growing, a thunderstorm, or a night sky filled with stars—can help you get in touch with the perfection that is inside of you. Get yourself mentally psyched for birth by facing challenges in your daily life with courage and confidence. Try not to complain too much. Learn to work through your discomforts and physical complaints without letting them completely overwhelm you. Learn to laugh. Try not to be a perfectionist; instead, learn to relax and "go with the flow." When you can do these things during your pregnancy, you will have developed important skills that will help you rise to the powerful occasion of labor and birth. I strongly believe that babies born to mothers who are confident about their bodies will also be confident. This is a powerful gift to give to our children.

You learned to follow your intuition and stay aware of your body's messages during pregnancy, and there's no reason to stop during labor, regardless of the place of birth. This is your right. Studies indicate that women who are allowed to eat, move about freely, and enjoy the company of supportive friends and family during labor are more likely to experience an uncomplicated labor and birth. Pay attention to what your body is telling you, and you will be guided to a healthy and fulfilling experience.

Breathing techniques that get you to focus on achieving a relaxed rhythm of inhalation and exhalation, rather than a series of practiced and forced breaths, will enable you to get through one contraction at a time while still providing ample oxygen to both you and the baby. Use techniques that focus on the opening of your body for the birth of your baby. Visual imagery during contractions, such as imagining that your cervix is an ever-widening circle of ripples on a still pond or a flower bud opening, can be comforting while your labor progresses. Practices that employ fixed breathing techniques for the various stages of labor can cause you to become exhausted and hyperventilated, as well as distract you from paying attention to your body as you try to force your attention onto the exercises. Since fixed breathing routines don't work for everyone, you may feel defeated if, for all your huffs and puffs, labor is still painful.

Birth is the combined physiological effort of both mother and baby. A baby who feels secure in getting born may make more of an effort to do so. This is not to say that babies that are harder to birth are unloved. When thinking about the birth, take the time to look closely and honestly at any ambivalent feelings you may have toward the baby or about being a parent, and think about how you might be relaying those feelings to your baby.

A recent article in a midwifery magazine (*Birth Gazette*, Summer 1995) discussed one midwife's observation that many babies appear to go through what she describes as a "spiritual emergency" during birth. Sometimes the baby takes a long time to be born, and sometimes immediately after birth the baby will be apathetic or even limp and without breath. Her theory is that these babies have a difficult start because they sense that their parents aren't fully welcoming them or because they are reluctant to face the experience of extrauterine life. Her solution, which she has found effective, is to speak warm and welcoming words to the baby immediately after birth and to have the parents do the same. This theory can be extended to the labor itself. We know that babies in the womb can hear and are affected by our voices and the emotional ambiance that surrounds them, so warm and welcoming words spoken to the baby during labor may well facilitate a smoother birth experience for both mother and child.

Focusing your love on your baby during labor is a healthy way to move the process along and is as effective as any breathing technique for helping you concentrate on opening your body to birth. Coupled with deep, natural breathing, it gives you an excellent tool for working with your labor.

Don't judge yourself during labor. Many women set standards for how they should behave during labor. Some feel that they should be very quiet; others feel that if they are practicing their relaxation exercises properly, then they will not feel any pain. Truthfully, there can be no set rules for birth other than that you must give it your best. Because birth is so spontaneous and unpredictable, flexibility within yourself is a wonderful attribute to foster. Try to tune in to what you feel and need as often as you can, and go with that. Allow yourself to act spontaneously, and you will be in harmony with your labor and birth needs. For example, if you feel the need to be very loud, allow yourself to release tension through your throat and voice by saying, "Open" in a deep, throaty tone. What you can best do to prepare for birth is regularly affirm your strength and ability to birth naturally, and then surrender to the experience.

❖ CARE OF THE MOTHER AFTER BIRTH ❖

The care and nurturing a woman gives to herself and receives from others in the days and months after she has given birth can greatly influence both her health and that of her baby. A woman may think that because the pregnancy is over and the baby is no longer so directly affected by her actions, she needn't care for herself as well. This is not true. Even if the birth was fairly easy, we must give ourselves the time to heal from the work of pregnancy and birth. We also have to do the formidable work of caring for a newborn and then a young child. There are sleepless nights; a child to be carried, rocked, bounced, and played with; and perhaps older children, housework, a job outside the home, and whatever else demands a mother's attention. Even the most supportive mate is not likely to put out the kind of full-time energy demanded of a mother. And even the seemingly automatic production of milk from our breasts requires us to be well rested and nourished.

Babies are totally dependent upon us, both physically *and* emotionally. They are visibly affected by our moods and health. Breast-feeding babies are also affected by the foods we eat and our emotional and mental states when we are nursing them. Some anthropologists actually consider the months after birth to be an extension of pregnancy. Consider the words of Ashley Montagu in *Growing Young* (1981): "The human when born has completed only half its gestation, the other half having to be completed outside the womb." Basically, the baby should be cared for in a manner that as closely as possible resembles the intimacy of pregnancy until this "exterogestation" is complete, which occurs, believe it or not, when the child begins crawling! Sleeping with your baby, carrying your baby in your arms or in a baby sling, and frequent breast-feeding provide this extended nurturing experience.

A well-cared-for new mother will have the best reserves for caring optimally for her baby. And every woman deserves to receive optimal care to ensure her own long-term health and happiness. It is well documented that women worldwide have developed practices commonly referred to as "mothering the mother." These practices take many forms, but where they exist, the new mother is generally free to stay in bed and rest, relax, establish her milk supply, and focus on her newborn for a variable amount of time (three weeks on average) while members of the community and family (generally other females) tend to her daily responsibilities.

Women in our society receive little special attention beyond a couple of days after the birth, when people come to "get a peek" at the baby. Yet this care and attention is vital, not only for our rest and recuperation, but also for our sense of worth. The validation coming from the feeling that what we are doing is important and challenging is critical to our desire to be mothers, especially in a culture that so frequently minimizes nurturing and mothering responsibilities. It is from a sense of self-worth that we offer the best care to our children and can feel the greatest joy with them.

The most likely way to get the support you need after giving birth is to ask for it. Arrange to take at least two months off from your job. Perhaps you can even take an extended leave while your child is young. Also, fathers should take off as much time as possible to nurture their new family. Babies like to get to know dads, too, and dad is the person from whom mom will likely feel the most comfortable receiving personal care. If the father cannot get off work for an extended period, perhaps a relative or close friend can assist the mother for a few weeks when he returns to work. If finances permit, you can hire a *doula*, a woman professionally trained to "mother the mother." Doula services are available in many parts of the United States, and a national organization trains and certifies them (see "Resources"). Whoever comes to help, let them play with the older children, tend to the housekeeping and meals, and run errands while you tend to yourself and the baby. Getting someone to help lessens the likelihood of your doing more than you need to either physically or emotionally, and it enables you to spend precious time with your newborn as she changes and grows before your eyes.

❖ HERBAL ALLIES FOR THE POSTPARTUM ❖

Herbs are an indispensable addition to a mother's postpartum wellness and recovery. They can be used for nearly every postpartum problem: soothing and healing a sore bottom, reducing hemorrhoids, promoting breast-milk production, healing nursing-related breast problems, and for soothing jangled nerves and emotions. The following are some basic guidelines; if you wish additional information, refer to "Further Reading."

Mother's Milk Tea I (see recipe under "Insufficient Milk Production," below) is an excellent drink for the days following birth. It promotes general relaxation, digestive comfort, and helps the mother weather the emotional storm that intense hormonal changes tend to stimulate. It also eases after-birth cramps.

Another great formula for emotional well-being during this time is Women's Balancing Blend, created by Rosemary Gladstar Slick. It is available through Mountain Rose Herbs (see "Resources") or can be prepared at home by mixing 1/2 ounce each of red raspberry leaves, strawberry leaves, peppermint, nettles, oatstraw, chrysanthemum flowers, and chamomile flowers, and 1/4 ounce each of horsetail, ginger root, dandelion leaves, and rose petals. Steep 1 tablespoon of the blend in 1 cup boiling water for twenty minutes, or use 1 handful per quart jar of water. Drink up to 6 cups a day, plain or sweetened. It's delicious!

Other herbs that you take internally to promote recovery and strength after birth are false unicorn root (use the tincture), a uterine tonic; comfrey leaf, which aids in the repair of any tissue damage; shepherd's purse, which allays bleeding; and nettles, which replenishes nutrients and helps balance blood sugar.

Herbal baths are sure promoters of postpartum healing and comfort. Useful for the reduction of soreness in the perineal area, as well as the healing of tears and stitches, hemorrhoids, and swelling, they are relaxing and antiseptic. They should be warm and at the mom's hip level.

Babies can accompany mothers in herbal baths, which promote the healing of the baby's umbilical site (thoroughly pat the area dry after the bath). In fact, newborns tend to love baths, probably because of their recent life spent in water. Moms (and dads) who take their newborns into baths can enjoy the special privilege of watching them relax and experience the bliss that a tub of warm water evokes.

Both of the following baths are prepared the same way: The bathtub should be very clean before the mother gets into it. The herbs are prepared as for standard infusions.

Herbal Bath I	*Herbal Bath II*
1 ounce comfrey leaves and root	2 ounces comfrey leaves
1 ounce blue cohosh	1 ounce calendula flowers
3/4 ounce shepherd's purse	1 ounce lavender flowers
1 ounce uva ursi	1 ounce sage
1 large, fresh garlic bulb	1/2 ounce myrrh
1/2 cup sea salt	3/4 cup sea salt

For Herbal Bath I, peel all the garlic cloves, place them in your blender with 2 cups water (any temperature is fine), blend at a high speed, and strain the resulting liquid into the tub. For both recipes, add the sea salt directly to the bath. Baths may be taken more than once a day, but at least once daily is optimal in the first week after birth. If for some reason you are unable to take baths, use hot compresses of these herbs (omitting the garlic and sea salt).

❖ BONDING AND BREAST-FEEDING: KEEPING THE CONNECTION STRONG ❖

BONDING

Bonding is not just what a super-glue does. It is also the incredibly warm and emotional melting in love that can occur when parent and child see each other for the first time. The term was first coined by some well-known physicians who recognized the importance of this process and popularized the concept. Clinically speaking, it refers to the idea that human mothers and fathers develop an optimal nurturing relationship with their children given the opportunity for immediate and sustained contact at birth.

The problem is that immediate bonding has become *expected* in the birthing process. Countless women today analyze the quality of their first interactions with their babies rather than allowing themselves to spontaneously explore and connect with them. Women who judge their initial interactions and reactions as inadequate may feel that they are doomed to a failed relationship with their children because bonding did not immediately take place. Indeed, professionals themselves may consider the parent-child relationship at risk if a woman expresses even the slightest hesitation or anxiety at the first sight of her child. Considering what she has just been through, a mother may well need a little time to recover and recognize the baby as her own. This is perfectly fine and normal, and certainly no cause for judgment from the doctor, midwife, or dad. Give mom a little time and some support, and the magic will happen.

Bonding also is love that begins before birth. It can occur beyond the mother-child relationship and in the child's relationships with siblings and others in the intimate circle of family and friends. Nor is it an experience limited to birth. Bonding can happen at any time in a parent-child relationship. People become deeply attached to each other when they share intimacy and when they open their hearts to each other. Adoptive mothers build unbreakable bonds with their children, even without the experience of immediate contact at birth. While birth is an experience that is ripe for depth of emotion and ease of openheartedness, separation at birth, while not desirable, may occasionally be necessary for medical care. This in no way does permanent damage to your relationship with your baby. If you determine that your baby needs medical care, then that is a loving choice, and any "damage" is repairable.

In the past couple of generations hospital policy has separated women from their babies at birth, overlooking their desires to see, touch, warm, and nurse their newborns. Babies are whisked to isolettes, placed under artificial lights for warmth, prodded, poked, examined, and "stabilized." Because most newborns are perfectly normal and healthy, this is totally unnecessary and, in my opinion, harmful, not to the experience of bonding, but to the parents' confidence in their ability to care for and protect their children. Lack of confidence in caring for one's own child is perhaps one of the greatest barriers to a healthy parent-child relationship.

It is within the magic of the mother-child relationship to be inextricably connected. Many mothers have the experience, for example, of waking in the night from the sensation of their milk letting down, just moments before their children wake from sleep hungry and looking for the breast to suckle. Through biology (literally "the word of life") we are connected to our babies. Biology is a very spiritual thing. The workings of our bodies are an intricate web influenced by and part of the physical and spiritual forces in the world. The more we tune in to this cellular level of communication (no, I am not referring to cellular telephones), the more we can begin to deliberately access it. But like interference on a telephone, the medical system's way of managing birth interferes with our ability to perceive messages and signals. It is our responsibility to clear the airways, stay away from high interference areas whenever possible, and then turn up our receivers and transmitters and listen closely. We can tune in to that wise place within us where we trust ourselves to know that our children are normal and healthy and that we will respond if they need help.

In the past twenty years, hospitals have made changes in their maternity wards primarily because mothers who were dissatisfied with their birth experience recognized the importance of immediate bonding and demanded greater freedom and choice in childbirth. Immediate mother-child contact, while popularized by physicians who researched the consequences of separation of the newborn and mother at birth, doesn't need to be "taught" to us; we just need not to be separated from our babies. A few of us may need some encouragement, but mostly we need to be in an environment that supports our abilities as parents and affords us the privacy to unite with our babies. We need to birth in environments that foster trust in birth, in the perfect physiology of human bodies, and in nature, rather than environments that see control and domination of birth as necessary to ensure health and survival. Love is the fruit surrounding the seed of instinct. Our love for our babies will guide us to make wise choices.

On a purely physical level, the immediate connection between a mother and her baby at birth serves certain biological imperatives. The sight, sound, and smell of your newborn and the nuzzling of your child to your breast (even if she doesn't immediately nurse) stimulate the release of powerful hormones causing your uterus to contract. This causes your uterine blood vessels to become constricted, preventing hemorrhage. (Hospitals frequently take away the baby and give the mother a synthetic hormone through injection or intravenous line to mimic the natural physiological process.) In addition, these sensory experiences inform the baby in a clear way who his or her mama is. While we no longer consciously depend on knowing our mother's scent in order to survive, as would a deer or other animal, this primal knowledge may be a significant part of our brain development, and lack of this stimulus may lead to developmental delays in ways yet unknown to us.

BREAST-FEEDING

The benefits of breast-feeding are innumerable. Researchers are just beginning to document increased immune response and enhanced intellectual potential in breast-fed babies. If we place our trust in our bodies and in nature, then it is logical to assume that our breasts produce milk after we give birth for important reasons.

The trend in bottle-feeding in the past few generations can be directly linked to economic motives from both the public and private sectors. Prior to World War II, babies were almost always breast-fed. But during the war, so many men had to leave the workforce to join the army that women were required to take their place in order to keep the economy functioning and to serve the war effort. As women left the home, bottle-feeding became more common. Around the same time, the newly founded bottle-feeding industry and many physicians promoted the notion that babies could not grow adequately on breast milk. My husband's grandmother often told me the story of how her doctor "made her" weigh her son (my father-in-law) before breast-feeding him, then again immediately after he nursed. If he did not gain a prescribed amount of ounces in a feeding, she was to supplement him with formula. Of course, with such a routine and with such doubt cast over her ability to adequately nourish her son at her breast, nursing did not last long. This is not an uncommon story.

Since World War II, billions of dollars have been made in the production of formula and other feeding paraphernalia—"the necessities of motherhood"—and the industry continues to grow. Hospitals receive thousands of dollars from formula makers for the endorsement of their brands. We have been brainwashed into believing that food from a cow, put into a can and bought in a store, is better for our babies than the milk from our own breasts, which is free!

Mothers will continue to make up a large percentage of the workforce, both out of necessity and out of a desire to be engaged in work outside of the home, but today breast-feeding is not just for stay-at-home mothers. La Leche League International (see your phone directory under "La Leche League" for local group leaders, or call 800-638-6607 for referrals worldwide) provides breast-feeding information and support for mothers with jobs that take them out of the home.

Because so much information on breast-feeding is available, I will not list all of its benefits here. But I do consider it such an important boost to a child's health that I am including herbal remedies for a few common problems to encourage you not to quit if you run into minor difficulties. Of course, not all women can breast-feed. Women who have had radical mastectomies will not be able to, nor can women who have undergone certain types of breast reductions and enlargements or who have active tuberculosis and certain other infectious diseases. My prayers go out to you to love yourself and know that you can still nourish (which at its root means "to suckle") your baby in many other ways. La Leche League can assist you in learning the many tricks available for solving breast-feeding problems and finding alternatives to breast-feeding.

KEEPING THE CONNECTION STRONG

Earlier in this chapter I mentioned the concept of exterogestation, the belief that a human baby continues the process of gestation outside the mother's womb. Allowed the continued closeness that uterine life provided, baby may develop many faculties, such as enhanced brain development as well as community orientation and a sense of belonging (and its attendant confidence and self-esteem) more fully than a baby who does not have prolonged and extensive physical contact and nurturing during (at least) the first postpartum year.

There are two child-rearing commonalities found in most tribal cultures, in addition to extended breast-feeding, that we have virtually excluded from our culture that allow for the experience of exterogestation to occur: "wearing" our children, and the family bed. In almost every society one could research, babies and young children are carried about in slings or packs, usually by their mothers, and sometimes by fathers or older siblings. Likewise, all over the globe, with the exception of many European countries, families sleep in the same bed, or at least in the same room. Cultures in which these practices occur, such as among the Pygmies or the !Kung bush people, both in Africa, tend to have a high degree of community orientation and cooperativeness among tribal members. These values are considered essential for the survival of the community. Our culture places greater emphasis on individuality, independence, and competition than on interdependence. Furthermore, sexuality in our society is a very confused issue to the point that having one's children sleep in the same bed or even in the same room, aside from an occasional experience if a child is ill or has had a nightmare, is considered by many to be sexually inappropriate.

These values and ideas are unfortunate for both parents and children. Children lose the warmth and security that comes from the experience of being held for much of the day and from sleeping in a family bed. Left to spend many hours in a crib or playpen, a baby misses the stimulation and experiential opportunities to be gained from being carried in a pack on mother's back or belly, or in a sling on her or dad's side. Studies have suggested that the act of co-sleeping may actually prevent sudden infant death syndrome (SIDS) as the parents' movements and breathing patterns may prevent a baby from lapsing into an apneic (nonbreathing) sleep pattern, from which, in the case of SIDS, a baby doesn't recover breathing and dies. While this suggestion is not conclusive, it is certainly thought-provoking. It is also infinitely more convenient for a nursing mother to have her baby tucked in near her in bed than to have to get up during the night to feed her baby.

The most common argument I hear against the family bed is that children will be spoiled and overdependent if allowed such ongoing closeness to mom and dad. Years ago I read a quote that I firmly believe. It said that children, like ripe fruit, only spoil if left on a shelf and forgotten. And I also believe that in our fervor to create fiercely independent children, we have labeled normal human dependence and need for interaction and connection as a pathological problem of overdependence. None of the families I know who have enjoyed the closeness of the family bed have raised children who exhibit unhealthy or neurotic behavior. In fact, most seem to be confident, healthy individuals with a beautiful sense of belonging to a family. The main inconvenience is that the parents need to be more creative in finding privacy and intimacy, an obstacle that is easily overcome.

From their earliest ages, my children have watched me cook, clean, sew, garden, harvest herbs, even midwife a few babies, from their perch on my back or hip! Recently, a midwife friend returned from Ghana with a gift for me, a small doll representing a Ghanaian midwife. The doll has one baby in her arms, presumably a newborn, and another in a pack on her back—presumably her child as well. In addition to the preciousness of being so connected to their babies and young children, parents who wear their babies gain the convenience of being able to go about their business without wondering what their babies are doing. Babies carried about in slings are easily comforted and, because they feel secure, are likely to be more content and even quieter than babies kept at a distance from parents when placed in a stroller. I have been able to keep my baby content at weddings and meetings (and births!) while he or she has been in the pack. Teething or colicky babies are frequently comforted by a walk in a sling or carrier, providing a simple home remedy for these common complaints that leave many parents feeling like they're getting a few grey hairs.

There are many types of packs available from a variety of sources ranging from Toys 'R Us and Sears to baby stores and baby catalogs. Over-the-shoulder carriers are ideal for newborns and convenient for carrying older children, while backpacks are great for carrying kids ranging from about five months old until about two-and-a-half years. The latter allow parents to have both hands completely free. The former allow mom to conveniently and discreetly nurse the baby. I have used a simple piece of long fabric with a knot tied over my shoulder as my sling, but there are soft and padded slings available in beautiful fabrics. If you choose a backpack for your older baby or child, find one with hip straps, allowing you to distribute some of the baby's weight onto your hips rather than only on your shoulders, to avoid back, neck, and shoulder strain.

❖ HERBAL ALLIES FOR COMMON BREAST-FEEDING PROBLEMS ❖

While breast-feeding is a process that our bodies are perfectly designed for, minor difficulties are common, particularly when a mother is establishing a nursing relationship with her first child. Most of us lack the support of mothers who breast-fed, because the past couple of generations in modernized countries have primarily used formula. Don't be too hard on yourself if you have some trouble; you are clearing a path that few have traveled for years, and it has become overgrown with brambles.

The herbal remedies listed below are safe for use when you are breast-feeding. The baby may get some of the herbs through your milk, but they are not harmful. Nevertheless, avoid highly stimulating herbs, herbs that strongly affect the hormones, cathartic herbs, and strongly narcotic herbs, all of which can cause undesirable side effects in your baby. If you are using an herbal remedy while breast-feeding and notice any side effects in your baby, reduce the strength of your preparation or discontinue it altogether.

INSUFFICIENT MILK PRODUCTION

Perhaps one of the most common reasons that discourages women from nursing is that they worry that they are not producing enough milk. This, however, is rarely the case with women who are eating well, drinking enough fluids, and allowing the baby to nurse often. Even if milk production *is* low, it can be increased by providing the mother with added nourishment and care. A baby who is gaining adequate weight is certainly getting enough milk, and, in general, so is a baby who is wetting six to eight diapers a day and pooping some too.

To increase your milk supply:

- Be sure to drink at least a half gallon of fluids a day: water, herbal tea (noncaffeinated), fresh fruit and vegetable juices, or soup broth. You need adequate fluids to produce adequate milk. When you aren't drinking enough, you are more likely to get depressed and fatigued; so keep a glass of water nearby to sip on.
- You also need adequate caloric intake (even more than during pregnancy!) as well as nutrients. Basically, your diet needs to be as healthy as a pregnancy diet with slightly less emphasis on protein and a greater emphasis on complex carbohydrates. Be sure to continue to eat calcium- and iron-rich foods so that you maintain the integrity of your body as you continue to grow your baby's body.
- Certain foods have a reputation for encouraging milk production. These include barley, oats, beets, carrots (especially carrot juice), winter squash, almonds, avocados, brown rice (and mochi, a Chinese ricecake available in natural-food stores) leafy greens, and sea vegetables (dulse, hijiki, and Kombu in particular). Thick, grain-based soups and porridges are used throughout the world to encourage more milk.

- Mother's Milk Tea is my all-time favorite tea for new moms and babies. This is a tasty tea you'll always want to keep on hand. It has many uses, including relief of indigestion for those of any age, stress, labor pains, postpartum cramps, aches, fevers, and "PMS," and it makes a nice herbal bath. Because it encourages restfulness, it's a great bedtime tea and nerve tonic for toddlers. Two versions are included in this book. Mother's Milk Tea I, described below, stimulates production of milk (herbs that do this are called "galactogogues"). Try making up a batch of the dried herbs late in your pregnancy. Nursing mothers can drink up to a quart a day. A slightly different version, described in "Colic (or the Sunset Blues)" in Chapter 6, eases this problem when taken by either mom or child and is especially useful for calming the nerves.

  To make Mother's Milk Tea, mix together the following dried herbs: 1 ounce chamomile flowers, 1 ounce catnip, 1/4 ounce fennel seeds, 1/2 ounce borage, and 1/8 ounce lavender flowers. To prepare the tea as a simple beverage, steep 1 tablespoon of the dried herbs in 1 cup boiling water for ten minutes; to prepare medicinally to increase milk, steep 1 handful in a quart jar of boiling water for twenty minutes and drink plenty!

- *Galax* means "milk," as in our *galaxy*, the Milky Way. The following herbs are more examples of galactogogues, herbs that increase milk production: blessed thistle, marshmallow root, slippery elm bark, dandelion root and leaves (the latter can also be eaten as cooked greens or in salads), nettles, alfalfa, red raspberry leaves, and oatstraw. Most of these can also be used to lift melancholy and mild depression, and they also improve the nutrient quality of your milk. They can be taken in infusions or tinctures in average doses of 1/2 to 1 ounce of dried herbs per quart of water, or 10 to 30 drops of tincture two to four times daily.

- Many times, what seems to be lack of milk is actually just an inhibition in the mother. Most of us did not grow up seeing women nursing babies, and we live in a culture that considers breasts as sex objects to be covered (except, of course, in certain magazines and advertisements). As a result, you may feel uncomfortable with the pleasurable sensuality of nursing your baby or with nursing in public. If these are problematic issues for you, speak with other women who have breast-fed and seek the support of La Leche League. There are many discreet methods of breast-feeding, and many public places have lounges or quiet areas where mothers can nurse in private. My personal belief is that letting people see what you are doing is a political act of the utmost importance if we are going to change societal views not only about breast-feeding, but also women's bodies.

Herbs can help you relax if you feel uptight when you nurse. Herbs such as chamomile, catnip, hops, lemon balm, and lavender gently soothe body and spirit, enabling you to slow down and tranquilly as feed your baby. Drink pleasant infusions sweetened lightly.

- Beer is an old wives' brew for increasing milk supply. It is high in calories, which help increase the amount of milk you produce, and the hops in beer, as well as the alcohol, encourage you to relax. This helps you to "let down" your milk, the process that lets the milk flow out of your breasts. Nonalcoholic beers, now available at many shops, provide the same benefits.

SORE NIPPLES

Sore nipples are the bane of breast-feeding. To have such tender tissue become sore and cracked is painful and very discouraging, especially for first-time moms getting started in their nursing relationship. Some soreness in the first few days after birth is pretty normal and common. After a short time, your nipples will toughen up and no longer be sore. Sometimes improper positioning of the baby on your nipple can lead to soreness. The baby's mouth should surround the nipple and much of the areola (the dark part), not just hang off the end of your breast. If you suspect this is the cause of your troubles and need help correcting the baby's placement, contact a local breast-feeding support group or experienced nursing mom.

Another common cause of sore nipples is thrush. This is a yeast infection on your nipples that is coming from the baby's mouth or has developed from wearing bras or nipple shields that cut off air circulation and prevent your nipples from staying sufficiently dry. Discontinue the use of shields and, if possible, go braless until the infection heals; otherwise, change bras every day. When your bra or shirt is wet, change to a dry one. You will notice that a thrush infection stays pretty damp and may even look weepy. Getting rid of it with just comfort measures such as salve is hard and it is likely to itch as well as feel sore. Refer to "Thrush" in Chapter 7 for treatment in addition to the following recommendations.

To soothe sore nipples:

- For cracked, dry, red nipples, regularly apply herbal salve made with comfrey root and calendula until your nipples become moisturized and heal.

- Use cocoa butter, almond oil, vitamin E, or lanolin on your nipples. Some folks are allergic to lanolin, so discontinue its use if you notice a reaction. Wipe off any residue before you nurse your baby.
- Aloe vera gel applied to your nipple brings cooling relief and helps heal cracks and cuts. It is intensely bitter, so you may need to rinse your nipples before nursing.
- Expose your nipples to fresh air and sunlight, or at least the latter, for a minimum of twenty minutes a day. If cold or privacy are problems, sunlight coming in through the window is adequate.
- If your nipples are painfully sore when you feed your baby, try nursing on one side for a day while you treat the other; then switch sides. This will not interfere with nursing and may give your nipples the needed time to heal.

PLUGGED DUCTS AND MASTITIS

Milk flows through ducts, little channels in your breasts, before it exits through your nipples. These channels can become blocked when they become engorged with milk or from physical constriction, which can occur from sleeping the wrong way or from wearing a too-snug bra.

Plugged ducts can become inflamed quickly and unexpectedly, causing severe discomfort. Some localized discomfort, a hard red knot, or streaky red area on your breast where the discomfort is centered are the first symptoms you're likely to notice. Fever, chills, malaise, dizziness, nausea, and general flu symptoms will then follow. This condition is commonly referred to as "mastitis," or breast infection. It is quite preventable, and if caught early, it can usually be cleared within twenty-four hours. Untreated, it can eventually lead to a breast abscess with a more serious systemic infection. Don't let it go that far!

Mothers who are very active or overtired are especially likely to develop mastitis. Perhaps this is because they are not settling down long enough to nurse the baby until the breasts are emptied or because fatigue lowers overall immunity. Plugged ducts are even more apt to occur when moms are not consuming enough fluids and healthy meals. If you've been overdoing it, slow down! If you notice any of the signs of breast inflammation, *stop everything!* Put on loose, warm, comfortable clothing; jump into bed or relax in a cozy chair with your baby and a cup of hot tea or broth; and observe all treatment recommendations that apply to you.

Discuss any fever or infection that occurs within the first weeks after birth with your health care provider. If accompanied by abdominal tenderness or foul-smelling vaginal discharge, this could be a uterine infection (childbed fever), which is very dangerous for the mother. You need to seek help immediately.

To treat mastitis:

- Rest, fluids, and nourishment, along with frequent nursing of the baby on the affected side, are the primary treatments for a plugged duct as well as the best prevention for and cure of mastitis. With the following suggestions you should notice improvement in six to twelve hours and complete recovery within twenty-four hours. You may notice slight discomfort (a sore or bruised feeling) for slightly longer. If you do, continue the internal remedies until you are completely well.
- Drink a tall glass of water (warm or at room temperature) every waking hour of your day. This is incredibly important! Sip on catnip tea to ease stress, tension, and discomfort.
- Eat very well, especially hearty grain and vegetable soups. Miso paste, made from soybeans, is particularly nourishing and is a beneficial addition to any soup stock.
- Take naps throughout the day. Have no visitors or social activities until you are completely recovered. If you relapse into fatigue, the problem can easily recur.
- Nurse your baby often *on the affected side* in order to drain the ducts thoroughly and to flush the breast. It may feel uncomfortable to suckle the baby on the painful breast, but doing so will shorten the duration of the blockage. Nursing the baby on the side with the infection is perfectly safe. However, if an abscess occurs anywhere near the nipple, nurse on the other breast and hand-express from the affected side.
- Use compresses and tub soaks to apply moist heat to your breasts. You can fill a sink or basin with hot water and hang your breast into it as you *gently* massage the blockage toward the nipple. Ginger root, chamomile, marshmallow root, burdock root, and slippery elm infusions can be used as compresses. Hot water will suffice if nothing else is available.
- Apply a poultice of freshly grated potato (just a regular baker or boiler will do) two to three times a day. This is a wonderful remedy because nearly everyone has a potato, and it is remarkably effective in reducing pain, blockage, and inflammation. Remove the poultice when it becomes warm, usually after about twenty minutes.
- Take 1 dropper of echinacea tincture every two to four hours depending on the severity of the problem. Continue for at least twenty-four hours after all signs of illness are past.

- Take 500 milligrams of vitamin C every two to four hours. You may notice that your baby's poops become looser, but this is of no concern.
- If you have a fever, drink *hot* elder blossom and peppermint infusion (1/2 ounce of each herb steeped for twenty minutes in a quart of boiling water). Keep drinking it until you break a sweat, up to 2 quarts. Stay warm under the covers.
- Should an abscess occur, follow instructions under "Abscesses" in Chapter 9. Many abscesses can be treated at home, but in serious instances you should consult an experienced health care practitioner.

As you move out of the realm of pregnancy and birth and begin caring for your newborn, I hope you will bring with you the knowledge that just as you were capable of bringing forth the life of your child, you are also capable of caring for him or her. Using the various techniques you learned in this chapter, you will be able to approach the care of your child with a sense of confidence in yourselves as parents and trust in your ability to be attentive to your child's health care needs.

Chapter 6

❖

Your Healthy Newborn

Newborns are strong and fragile at the same time. They carry in their little bodies the mystery and magic of life, yet are totally dependent on us for support. Caring for a newborn calls for the parents to be patient and intuitive in learning the baby's signals. It would be so much easier if babies came with instructions.

Keeping your baby close to you will help you learn what he or she is asking for and help you develop your instincts. Thankfully, babies have simple desires and needs—mainly warmth, food, dryness, love, a bit of stimulation, and a lot of security. The challenge lies in learning to interpret their requests and to parent with confidence. This chapter will provide you with some basic information about what you can expect from a healthy newborn baby. You will learn about the baby's vital signs, how to interpret your baby's "language," and how to recognize when your baby is ill.

Before addressing the topic of newborn care, I want to acknowledge again the important connection between the health of the mother with that of her baby. A well-nourished mother has the greatest likelihood of birthing a healthy baby. Strong babies, likewise, have the greatest resilience. Habits such as cigarette smoking and drug use during pregnancy are clearly linked with prenatal and childhood health problems. There is greater likelihood of premature birth, low birth weight, developmental anomalies, and even respiratory problems in toddlers. On the other hand, babies born with an adequate birth weight (over 6 1/2 pounds) to mothers in good health are at the least risk for birth and childhood health problems.

In the same way that a healthy pregnant mother will usually have a healthy baby, health in a breast-feeding baby is directly related to the mom's well-being. Breast-feeding fortifies children against illness, but a woman must be in good health if she is going to provide nourishing milk to her child. When the baby is sick, working with the nursing mother's diet and giving herbal remedies directly to the mother will benefit the baby as well. In the pediatric philosophy of traditional Chinese medicine, the main approach to restoring health to an ill breast-feeding baby is to treat the mother. The connection between the wellness of the two is so linked that it is thought that indiscretions in the mother's lifestyle, such as eating overly rich foods, can cause illness in the baby. In fact, it is very common for a breast-feeding mother to eat certain foods and then notice soon after that her baby has become ill or uncomfortable. For example, a woman may eat a large bowl of ice cream and notice that her baby is congested the next day, or she may drink coffee and notice that her baby is fussy and unable to sleep that night.

Even when women don't breast-feed, their health affects their babies. If a mother doesn't take care of herself, she is more likely to become ill or exhausted. She will then be exposing the baby to her illness or, at the least, may be too tired to provide the baby with the care he or she needs. This is true of the father as well. The responsibility parents have can seem daunting, but we can choose to take pride in the great influence we have on our children through the examples we set. We can, from the start, influence them in a direction that teaches awareness between the actions we take and how they affect our wellness, and also how we affect others.

❖ YOUR BABY'S BODY ❖

APPEARANCE

Shortly after birth most babies have a slightly reddish appearance, which gradually fades to a nice pink over the first couple of days. For the first twenty-four hours, some babies have bluish hands and feet, which is frequently normal though you should mention it to your midwife or health care provider.

When the baby comes through the birth canal, the bones of the head overlap to a greater or lesser degree, depending upon the tightness of the fit and the length of time spent in the canal. This normal physiological process, known as "molding," gives some babies a "cone-head" appearance. After the first day the baby's head has usually assumed a nice round shape. Likewise, if the nose was pressed a bit flat at birth, it begins to perk up in the first postpartum days.

Newborns have an incredible purity about them down to the very smallest details of their beings. Their scent is indescribably fresh and sweet (the image that always comes to my mind is the scent of the air after a spring thundershower). Their eyes open wide and drink in all that they see with a totally receptive mind and nonjudging heart, speaking a million words without a sound. Their tiny fingers grasp and hold with firmness. If you spend an extra minute you can feel yourself melt into oneness with that child. Just to be in the presence of a newborn is magical. Their stillness when sleeping can bring peace to our busy minds as nothing else can.

Take the time to gaze into your baby's eyes, look at her toes, hold his hand, nuzzle closely to her head, and fill yourself with the scent of your child. You will begin a relationship that enables you to know your child deeply and closely, and this relationship will be the best guide to your child's health that you can ever have.

Regularly checking your baby's "vital signs" is unnecessary (except for temperature, which your midwife may want you to check a few times each day for the first few days after birth). But if you have any concerns about your baby's well-being, there are a few basics to consider.

TEMPERATURE

Every baby has his or her own rhythms and preferences, but some things are pretty standard. A newborn's temperature measured rectally averages about 98.6 degrees Fahrenheit. An easy, less-invasive alternative to rectal measurement is to put the tip of the thermometer in the baby's armpit and snuggle the baby's arm down against his side for five minutes. This is called the "axillary" temperature and is typically 1 degree lower than rectal measurement (so 97.6 degrees is normal).

Any newborn with an elevated temperature needs close attention, though it may be normal at 99 degrees Fahrenheit for the first twenty-four hours. Most often, the baby is overdressed or slightly dehydrated. Remove blankets and keep the baby in just a diaper and T-shirt if the room is warm. Recheck the baby's temperature after fifteen minutes. If it is still elevated, sponge the baby's wrists, feet, and forehead with tepid water (not cold!), and give the baby the breast or a bit of boiled water by eyedropper, providing liquid to drink until he'll take no more. If after an hour the temperature is still above normal, or if the baby shows signs of illness (see the end of this chapter), seek an experienced midwife or a physician immediately.

Babies need to be kept warm, not swelteringly hot. By touching the skin you can tell if your baby is too warm or cold. Generally the feet and hands should feel comfortably warm but slightly cooler than the chest and back. If the baby's hands feel quite warm, she may be overdressed or may be running a fever. Adjust the child's clothing and the room temperature accordingly; then check the baby's temperature.

A baby is usually a nice pink color. A baby who looks white and mottled or who has blue hands or feet may be chilled. A baby who appears ruddy may be too hot. These color changes may also indicate serious health concerns, so consult with your care provider if adjusting clothing and room temperature doesn't solve the problem.

BREATHING

A baby's breathing is often irregular, possibly with occasional lapses for up to twelve seconds. Babies may also take occasional little gulps of air. However, a baby's breathing should be effortless. There should be no grunting or wheezing sounds, and the chest should not heave. If your baby stops breathing for longer than twelve seconds, turns blue, or exhibits any of the signs of respiratory distress just mentioned, get immediate help. Your baby could have an infection or another problem that needs attention.

The normal breathing rate is usually about 30 to 40 breaths per minute. Sometimes the respiratory rate is up to 60 breaths a minute on the first day after birth. To compute the breathing rate, just listen closely and count how many breaths your baby takes in sixty seconds (use a watch or clock with a second hand as you count).

Babies commonly sneeze in the first couple of days after birth; this is how they clear their breathing passages. A tiny bit of rattling mucus in the nose will clear itself out with sneezes. Healthy newborns, however, do not have runny noses.

HEARTBEAT

To check your baby's heart rate, just put your fingers or ear over her heart and count the beats for one minute.

A healthy baby's heart rate averages between 110 and 150 beats each minute, fluctuating according to sleeping, nursing, and movement. A healthy baby may have a sleeping heart rate as low as 80 beats per minute. A baby whose heartbeat is well above or below this range may have a health problem, so speak with your midwife or physician promptly.

SLEEPING

Each newborn sleeps a varying amount depending on that child's personality, but most sleep for many hours at a time, waking for brief periods to nurse and make eye contact with you. Some newborns take naps for hours at a time, while others take short, frequent naps. Babies commonly and normally fall asleep shortly after being put to the breast to nurse. Many times they will continue to nurse during a nap.

There really is no rule about how much sleep is acceptable for newborns, but babies should have some alert and bright-eyed times each day and should be eager to nurse even if they doze while doing so. Physicians generally recommend that babies not be allowed to sleep more than four hours at a time during the day, for fear that they won't eat often enough if they sleep too much. In practice, I've found that babies usually wake to nurse or eat within this timeframe. If your baby is not showing signs of jaundice, infection, or general lethargy (see "Signs of Illness in the Newborn," at the end of this chapter), there is no harm in an occasional longer nap.

Much to the chagrin of their parents, some babies sleep very little. For unknown reasons, they take few naps or very short naps, keeping their parents on call for most of the day. While most babies will sleep a considerable amount during the first few days or even weeks after the birth, there are newborns who quickly kick the nap habit and want to nurse (or eat) and be held nearly all day. Fortunately, these babies often sleep well at night, though not always.

If you have such a baby, try to arrange for time each day, particularly in the first few months after the birth, when you can take a shower, nap, enjoy a decent meal, or replenish yourself however you need to in order to maintain your health (and sanity!). Be sure to relax when the baby does nap, and get to sleep early at night. Full-time parenting of a kid who doesn't sleep much, no matter how much you adore the child, can quickly become draining. If you take care of yourself well, you will have more energy for your high-needs baby. Eventually your baby will learn to sleep well through the night, but for the time being, develop your support system so you don't burn out. "Wearing" your baby in a sling or backpack can give you time with your hands free, while keeping baby happily occupied.

EATING

Some babies take a little while after birth to start nursing—even a few hours or more. How much a baby nurses will vary, but it is generally felt that a newborn should nurse at least every three to four hours. (I usually do not wake my babies just to nurse if they nurse with *enthusiasm* when they wake on their own.) Most newborns will nurse more often than that. If your baby is completely refusing your breast but has no health problems, then you will need to be patient but persistent in order to establish nursing. Given this, breast-feeding will usually begin within the first twenty-four hours. If not, seek the support of a La Leche League leader, a lactation consultant, or a health care worker such as your midwife, who can teach you how to express and feed the baby your milk via another route until the baby begins to suckle. This is necessary to prevent the baby from becoming dehydrated or hypoglycemic.

A listless, lethargic baby who does not want to nurse much is probably not feeling well and may have a condition that requires attention (see "Jaundice" and "General Infections in the Newborn" in Chapter 7).

It is fine to offer your breast to your baby whenever she cries or if you think she may be hungry. A baby will only suckle if she wants to; she'll push your nipple away with her lips if she doesn't want to nurse.

Spitting up is common and is probably just some overflow. To cut down on spitting up, feed your baby in a calm environment, letting yourself fully relax and hold the baby firmly and lovingly, without jiggling and bouncing. A baby with projectile vomiting (long-distance, forceful vomiting) needs further medical attention. If after you nurse your little one you pick him up with your hands around his belly, forcing his food back up, don't worry; that is not projectile vomiting.

Babies have unique nursing styles. Some nurse heartily for two-hour stretches; others take sips here and there. The frequency and amount of elimination is a good indication of whether your baby is eating enough, as is weight gain. Newborns begin to visibly fill out in the first days and weeks after birth.

ELIMINATION

A baby should urinate and have a bowel movement at least once in the first twenty-four hours after birth. After your milk comes in, the baby will usually wet a minimum of six diapers a day. For the first couple of days after birth, the baby's stools will be black and tarlike. These stools are called "meconium" and are what was in your baby's intestines before birth. After the first few days, the poops turn a golden brown color and have a loose consistency. Babies have unique bowel habits ranging anywhere from a few a day to a few over a couple of days. If your baby is not having a bowel movement at least every couple of days, you may want to look at your diet to rule out anything that could be constipating the baby. Common causes are dairy foods, peanut butter, wheat, and red meat.

CRYING

It's a fact of life that even the happiest babies sometimes cry, for one simple reason: Crying is the language of babies. A newborn cannot simply say, "My diaper is wet—will you please change it?" If you don't notice that your baby needs a diaper change, then after a while he will need to inform you. Crying is the most probable technique he'll use.

Some babies are more patient than others, and some parents are so incredibly attentive that their babies rarely cry. Breast-fed babies may actually cry less often than their bottle-fed counterparts because the relationship between mother and child tends to be very intimate and the moms quickly learn to respond to their babies' subtle messages. But even breast-fed babies fuss and cry. All children teethe, get overtired, have an occasional ache or fright, or experience some reason to become inconsolable at some point before they go off to college.

Since a fussy baby can be so trying on our patience, our task is to learn to masterfully comfort our kids when possible and even to let them cry for a bit if necessary without taking their unhappiness personally and without become so frustrated that we lash out at them. If you are holding your beautiful baby peacefully asleep in your arms at this moment, the idea of being irritated at such an angel may seem hard to imagine, but someday at four in the morning, pacing with a teething baby, perhaps you'll remember this page. Unfortunately, one of the most common reasons parents in child abuse cases give for battering their babies is that the baby just wouldn't stop crying. There is, of course, absolutely no excuse for abusing a child. You must learn how to cope.

If your baby is fussy, irritable, or even outright screaming, there are some basic steps you can take to try to comfort your baby without losing your cool. First, carefully look your baby over from head to toe to be certain that nothing obvious is causing physical discomfort. Even a hair that has become tightly wound around a finger or toe can cause extreme pain as well as endanger the circulation of that body part. Another possibility is that your baby has colic (see Chapter 7). If your baby doesn't seem to have any physical injuries, has no fever, normally does not get colic, and is fed, has a dry diaper, and isn't too hot or too cold, you can try to play with or rock him or her. Of course, if the baby is injured or seems sick, you will need to take the steps appropriate for that situation.

If the baby is fine but fussy despite your efforts to offer comfort and you are becoming irritated or exhausted, put the baby down somewhere safe and get some fresh air or go to a quiet place in your house for just a few minutes or as long as you need to gather your peace and composure. If you are harried, your baby will perceive this through your body language (smell, muscular tension, irritable behavior) and will resist settling down. When you feel at peace, return to your baby and try again to offer comfort. Don't hesitate to enlist your spouse, or call a relative, friend, or even a neighbor if you are a single parent and need support. "Wearing" your baby in a sling while you go about your business will give your baby a sense of closeness to you while allowing the baby to be gently rocked by the movement of mom or dad's body. You will feel less frustrated and your baby is likely to drop off to sleep.

❖ SIGNS OF ILLNESS IN THE NEWBORN ❖

Any baby who just "doesn't seem well" to the parents, particularly to the mom, should be evaluated by an experienced health care practitioner. Parents often have a keen sense of whether their children are well or ill.

If the baby is ill, consult with your midwife or physician to determine the best approach for healing. When you determine the cause of the problem, you can refer to the next chapter for appropriate treatment possibilities. No matter where or how you choose to heal your baby, your love and constant presence are his or her most important medicine. Talk to, touch, nurse, cuddle, and reassure your newborn.

WHEN TO SEEK MEDICAL CARE

Some signs of illness requiring the attention of a health care practitioner include: not wanting to nurse or eat; abnormal temperature; irritability combined with any of these signs; jaundice combined with any of these signs; bulging anterior fontanel (soft spot on baby's head); very stiff or floppy body; baby just "doesn't seem well."

BABIES IN NEED OF SPECIAL CARE

While it is beyond the scope of this book to provide information on caring for babies with severe congenital or health problems, it is important to me that these babies and their parents not feel left out of this discussion. Health is much more than the absence of illness. It is also a positive attitude in the face of illness, disability, or limitation. If your baby was born "different" from what you'd hoped or expected, please know that many support groups and loving people care deeply about children and can help you accept and learn to care for your child fully. Cascade Health Care Products has a parenting catalog called "Imprints" that contains a fine selection of reading materials and videos on dealing with pregnancy loss and "special babies." Midwives can frequently help you locate resources in your community.

Should your baby require medical care, you can usually stay with him or her. Most hospitals are now supportive of breast-feeding when possible and sometimes even give babies their mothers' milk through tubes if nursing by mouth is impossible. Spending time with your baby adds to the chances of your baby's recovery, particularly in the case of prematurity. Babies held and touched often are known to recover health and gain weight faster than those receiving minimal contact. If your baby is terminally ill, the contact you have will give you cherished memories to draw upon in the years to come; and while the experience of illness or loss of a child is incredibly painful, those memories will help you, in time, to feel a sense of completion with the experience.

Chapter 7

❖

Natural Remedies for Newborns and Babies

As babies adapt to life outside the womb, they undergo certain physiological changes to adapt to their new environment. As you will learn in this chapter, jaundice and even "colic" occur normally in response to a baby's body learning to function without the help of the placenta and the mother's circulation, which until birth provided all the baby's food and oxygen requirements and served as the baby's eliminatory system.

Babies also can develop health problems that range in severity from the very minor, such as diaper rash, to the serious, such as kernicterus, a complication of advanced jaundice. This chapter discusses commonly occurring health conditions in the most likely chronological order and provides complete information on how to prevent and naturally treat certain problems, as well as how to recognize when a baby needs medical care. You can also refer to Chapter 9, "Natural Remedies for Children's Complaints: An A–Z Guide" for general conditions such as colds, which are not discussed in this chapter.

❖ EYE CARE ❖

In the hospital, silver nitrate or other antibiotic drops are routinely put into a newborn's eyes. This practice was begun in 1884 as a treatment and prevention of gonorrheal infection, which in a baby's eyes can lead to blindness.

Silver nitrate is extremely burning and irritating, potentially harmful in itself. It causes the baby's eyes to swell closed, preventing initial eye contact between the baby and the parents. While most hospitals abandoned the use of silver nitrate about ten years ago, some do still use it, primarily because it is inexpensive. Be certain to ask what your hospital uses if that is where you are birthing. If you choose to use drops in your baby's eyes, an alternative antibiotic ointment is preferable and equally effective.

Many parents who are birthing at home and know they don't have gonorrhea choose not to treat their babies' eyes unless signs of infection develop. Some who wish to use a preventative squeeze a few drops of colostrum (the nutrient-rich liquid in the breasts before the milk comes in) into each of the baby's eyes because it contains natural antibiotics. Whether or not to treat a baby with prophylactic eye care is each parent's choice, and it should be an informed decision.

If infection develops and worsens despite your efforts to resolve it, or if a mild infection does not readily respond to home treatment, seek medical care and antibiotic treatment. Most often irritation of the newborn's eyes is a result of a plugged tear duct or yeast or other organism transmitted during a vaginal birth or from someone's fingers touching the baby's eye. Most such organisms are not dangerous.

In the event of gonorrhea, you have twenty-four hours from the onset of symptoms (red or runny eyes) to provide treatment before permanent damage results.

To treat eye irritations and infections:

- To treat a minor eye irritation or infection with discharge, redness, or swelling, use the following tea in addition to or instead of breast milk: Steep 1 tablespoon of chamomile blossoms and 1/8 teaspoon of goldenseal powder in 1/2 cup boiling water for twenty minutes. Strain twice. Clean the eyes every two hours with a fresh cloth or sterile gauze dipped in the tea. (Chamomile soothes and cools the inflammation; goldenseal is an antibiotic.)
- When you apply remedies to the baby's eyes, do not allow the infected eye to contaminate the clear one. Place your remedy into the inner corner of the infected eye and let it run outward. Always treat both eyes with different cloths. Wash or discard cloths after each use, and wash your hands well.
- If your baby has an eye infection, you can take 25 drops of echinacea tincture four times a day, some of which will pass through your breast milk to the baby. Nurse often. Give your baby an oral dose of 2 drops of echinacea tincture diluted in water (use an eyedropper) four times a day.

Blocked tear ducts can lead to irritation, swelling, and discharge but usually resolve themselves on their own within the first year. To encourage them to open, gently massage the area on the inside of the bridge of the nose and beneath the duct in a downward direction. Use cool chamomile tea compresses to soothe the area.

❖ CIRCUMCISION AND CARE OF THE PENIS ❖

Circumcision is the surgical removal of the protective skin covering the glans of the penis. During the procedure, baby boys are strapped to a restraining board, and the foreskin is spread open with a metal clamp and cut off with a knife. (When a baby is circumcised by a moyl, the person in the Jewish tradition trained and ordained to perform circumcision, he is not strapped down, and wine is used as an anesthetic.) The surgery can lead to infection, hemorrhage, permanent damage to the penis, and perhaps permanent psychological damage.

The medical and hygienic reasons given to justify circumcision are outdated and have generally been discredited. An uncircumcised penis, given proper care, will rarely become infected, stuck (a condition known as "phimosis"), or "dirty." In fact, the foreskin serves to protect the inner part of the penis from irritation.

I strongly encourage all couples who are pregnant and those with uncircumcised sons to read Anne Briggs' thorough and informative book *Circumcision: What Every Parent Should Know.* It includes historical and current facts about circumcision, describes the process in detail, and outlines the care of uncircumcised boys.

Even if your religious or social convictions lead you to circumcise, please remember that this is a surgical procedure that should be done with care for your child's health and with respect for his sensitivity to pain, which is certainly very real and fully functioning even in the first days of life. If you choose to have your baby circumcised rather than leave him intact, ask your practitioner to use a local anesthetic for the procedure. I also hope you will read Anne's book and reconsider whether circumcision is necessary.

WHEN TO SEEK MEDICAL CARE

Any bleeding or infections that occur in conjunction with a circumcision require the immediate care of a pediatrician. A newborn can experience serious problems should either infection or hemorrhage occur. These are rare but do happen, so educate yourself about what to expect after the procedure.

Until the child reaches age four, the uncircumcised penis needs no special attention other than the basic soap-and-water washing that the rest of the body receives. Never retract the foreskin for washing. Should irritation occur, the following will help:

- Rinse with warm water two or three times days daily; then apply one of the following directly onto the glans and over the foreskin: calendula oil, aloe vera gel; or a rinse made of echinacea and calendula tinctures (use 10 drops of each in 1/3 cup lukewarm water), or chickweed tea.

- For more severe irritations, give echinacea tincture, one-half of the baby's body weight in drops, internally three to four times a day, along with 250 milligrams of vitamin C each time.

For more information, see "Penis Irritations and Care" in Chapter 9.

❖ CARE OF THE UMBILICAL CORD ❖

If you keep your baby in a warm, dry room and keep the diapers folded beneath the stump of the umbilical cord, the cord will usually dry up and fall off within five to seven days of birth. Occasionally it will take longer.

Just before the cord falls off, you may notice a fleshy sort of smell coming from the bellybutton. The odor should not be foul; nor should you see any redness. When the cord falls off, the umbilicus (navel) may contain what appears to be pus but is actually just an open site that still requires healing. To differentiate the normal appearance of the open site from one that is infected, thoroughly clean the bellybutton with a cotton swab that has been dipped in rubbing alcohol.

Should you see any mild redness or wish to take prophylactic measures, use any of the following. If you see significant signs of infection, promptly seek medical help.

- Squeeze breast milk into the bellybutton every couple of hours. The antibodies in your breast milk challenge infections in your baby's body.
- Sprinkle goldenseal powder all over the umbilicus at each diaper change. It is drying in powder form and is also an antibiotic.
- Put a few drops of echinacea tincture onto the stump. The mother can take 35 drops of this tincture internally each day, or the baby can have a few drops twice a day. Let the baby suck the tincture out of the dropper as he or she sucks on your nipple.
- Bring your baby into your postpartum herbal bath. (Herbal baths are described in "Herbal Allies for the Postpartum" in Chapter 5.) Pat the baby's belly dry after each bath.

❖ GENERAL INFECTION IN THE NEWBORN ❖

Babies born at home are less likely to develop infections than are those born in a hospital. This is because home environments are less likely to harbor disease-causing bacteria and viruses, and because babies receive passive immunity through their mothers, who are accustomed to the organisms in the home. Infection can arise in any baby, however, and once it does, it needs to be recognized and attended to quickly. Healthy babies are resilient and possess a great deal of vital energy; a weak or sick baby can "go downhill" fast.

The best way to prevent infection in a newborn is to nurture and grow a strong, healthy baby during pregnancy. A healthy full-term baby is likely to have an optimally functioning immune system with peak resistance to illness. Excellent nutrition during pregnancy is one of the key factors in preventing prematurity, early rupture of the amniotic sac, and hypoglycemia (an abnormally low level of blood glucose), all of which increase the baby's susceptibility to infection. As stress can weaken immunity, keep the birth and postpartum environments as calm as possible. Avoid allowing sick people to visit your newborn during the first weeks. This may seem obvious, but people's desire to see and hold a newborn often overrides their common sense. (One friend brought her coughing and sneezing child to our home, along with a meal for us, a few days after our second baby was born.)

Prolonged broken waters (membranes) before birth and aspiration of meconium (the baby's prenatal stools) can also increase the risk of infection. A mother who has had an infection, such as vaginal strep during pregnancy, can pass it on to the baby. If you have been or currently are dealing with an infection, you need to carefully consider the risks and benefits of home and hospital birth for your baby.

WHEN TO SEEK MEDICAL HELP

Some signs of infection in the baby include: not wanting to nurse or eat; abnormal temperature; irritability combined with any of these signs; jaundice combined with any of these signs; bulging anterior fontanel (soft spot on baby's head); very stiff or floppy body; baby just "doesn't seem well."

If your baby is at risk for infection but seems totally well, plenty of nursing, loving care, and general awareness should be enough. Never underestimate the value of breast milk in healing infections. Colostrum and mother's milk are exceedingly rich in antibodies that stimulate and protect the newborn's immune system, enabling the child to overcome illness. In addition, the closeness and comfort your baby derives from nursing establishes health.

A newborn can have an elevated temperature and be irritable because he is overbundled or otherwise hot and is becoming dehydrated. Nurse the baby frequently and adjust room temperature and clothing accordingly. If the baby refuses to nurse, try giving dilute molasses water (1 tablespoon molasses to 1 cup boiled water) with an eyedropper and sponge the baby with tepid water. If you see no improvement within an hour, the baby may actually be ill.

If the baby is at risk for infection, the nursing mother can take 30 drops of echinacea tincture and 500 milligrams of vitamin C four times a day for five days after the birth. You can also give the baby 3 drops of echinacea tincture three times a day. Slip an eyedropper containing the drops into the baby's mouth next to your nipple as he or she nurses.

❖ Babies' Skin Care and Rashes ❖

Babies are born with a varying amount of "vernix," a creamy white substance, on their skin. Vernix is a nutrient-rich coating that covers the baby while in the womb and keeps the skin from getting "pruney" (how your fingers and toes get after too long in the bathtub). After birth it protects the baby's skin from dryness, irritation, and infection. Do not wash it off; massage it into your baby.

You don't need to wash a newborn with soap, but if you do use it choose one that is mild, pure, and unscented. Added perfumes can interfere with either you or your baby recognizing each other's natural scent. Clean off dried blood from the birth and meconium by rubbing with a little almond or olive oil. You can also massage these oils into the baby's skin, particularly around the ankles, hands, and feet to prevent peeling and cracking.

During the first few weeks, newborns may develop little white bumps on their noses and sometimes in other areas. Known as "milia," they are a normal response of the baby's oil glands and pores beginning to work. They will disappear on their own.

At some point your baby probably will have at least a mild diaper rash. The most common causes are disposable diapers, something the mother ate or drank that irritated her system, a yeast infection, going too long without a diaper change, teething, a reaction to laundry soap, or a cold.

If your baby's skin is dry and chafed, treat the rash by moistening and nourishing the skin. A healing salve that is excellent for baby's bottoms can be made from 1/2 ounce calendula flowers, 1 ounce fresh chickweed, 1/2 ounce comfrey leaves or root, 1/4 ounce chamomile flowers, 1/2 fresh plantain leaf, 1 pint olive oil (or more; use enough to cover herbs), and pure beeswax. A field guide can help you identify chickweed and plantain, both of which grow wild, even in the city. *Plantago major* is the preferable plantain to use, but lance-leaf (*Plantago lanceolata*) is also acceptable. See "Herbal Preparations" in Chapter 4 for full instructions on the preparation of salves.

Changing diapers as soon as they are wet or soiled and letting the baby go diaperless as often as possible prevents and cures diaper rash.

Exposing the little one's bottom to the sun for ten minutes a day is one of the best rash medicines you can find. Even sunlight coming though a window is adequate.

A red, sore, bumpy type of rash is often due to a yeast infection. See "Thrush," below, addressing this common problem.

A note about diapering: Disposable diapers, while a convenience for busy parents, are not the best option for either babies or the environment. Diaper rash occurs more often in babies who wear plastic diapers because their wetness is less noticeable and therefore they get changed less frequently than cloth-diapered babies. Disposable diapers contain bleach, traces of dioxin, and other chemicals that can lead to skin irritations. Both the plastic in diapers and the chemicals used to manufacture them pose environmental hazards. In addition, they contribute an enormous amount of waste to landfills. Harmful and resistant strains of infectious diseases including polio and hepatitis can incubate in the discarded diapers found in landfills, creating a threat to public health.

In the long run, cloth diapers cost less to use than disposables and pose minimal threat to the ecosystem. The extra effort in laundering them is worthwhile for your baby as well as generations to come.

❖ JAUNDICE ❖

A newborn who develops yellowish skin and eyes is considered to be jaundiced. There are three types of newborn jaundice: physiological, breast-milk, and pathological. While each form has its own cause, they all create a similar condition in the body: a greater abundance of red blood cells than the body can easily assimilate or eliminate. Physiological and breast-milk jaundice can almost always be resolved at home; however, untreated severe jaundice and pathological jaundice can lead to permanent brain damage. Read below to learn about the forms of jaundice, and seek experienced help if you are treating a jaundiced baby. Jaundice that is not responding to home care or a baby whose symptoms are worsening needs immediate medical attention.

PHYSIOLOGICAL JAUNDICE

A baby in the womb receives his or her entire supply of oxygen from red blood cells. Since the baby is not deriving oxygen from the air, a great supply of red blood cells (RBCs) is needed for oxygenation. When the baby is born and begins to breathe, he or she gets oxygen from the air and no longer needs so many RBCs. The excess RBCs need transformation and elimination. A byproduct of the transformation process is called "bilirubin." Bilirubin, which is yellow in color, can get backed up and reabsorbed, giving the skin the characteristic yellow color of jaundice. Physiological jaundice generally appears on the third day after birth, peaks on about the fourth day, and usually subsides by the sixth day after birth. If the baby seems otherwise healthy, the jaundice does not present a problem. In fact, some evidence indicates that jaundice is not only a natural response, but also one that protects a baby's cells from damage early in life.

If the bilirubin level is exceedingly high, the baby runs the risk of a disease called "kernicterus," which can lead to brain damage. Symptoms that indicate the disease may be developing include lethargy, excessive sleeping, poor nursing, irritability, high-pitched crying, poor muscle tone (floppy body), and vomiting. If any of these signs accompany the jaundice (or if your newborn seems sick at all), promptly seek experienced care.

Factors increasing the likelihood and risk of jaundice include premature birth; distress during labor or birth; and a mother who takes drugs or medications during pregnancy or labor or while breast-feeding. A baby who has a ruddy complexion at birth or during the first couple of days afterward may be more likely to develop jaundice, as is one given medications at birth.

Prevention is the best medicine here. Women who eat well and take excellent care of themselves during pregnancy have the best chance of birthing full-term babies with strong organs. These babies usually clear out RBCs effectively and have little, if any, jaundice and rarely any problems if jaundice does develop. A healthy diet includes herbs rich in nutrients and supportive of the mother's liver, which in turn helps to nurture and strengthen the baby. Alfalfa leaf (tea, tincture, or tablets), in conjunction with dandelion root and leaves (tea, tincture, or as a salad or cooked green) can be used throughout pregnancy to supplement iron and other minerals. Dandelion specifically supports and strengthens the liver and promotes healthy bowel function. Alfalfa, used moderately in late pregnancy, has many benefits. Most notably, it prevents hemorrhage in the mother and baby because it is high in vitamin K. Consequently, the mother can usually forego vitamin K injections (a routine hospital procedure), which in fact increase the likelihood of jaundice.

Immediate and frequent nursing encourages bowel movements and healthy intestinal flora and enzymes that enable your baby to eliminate bilirubin. Mothers should drink plenty of water and Mother's Milk Tea I (see "Insufficient Milk Production" in Chapter 5). Let your baby nurse often even if you have only colostrum in your breasts.

While some traditional cultures keep babies in darkness for up to three weeks after birth, some exposure to sunlight during the first week is advisable for preventing jaundice. After the first twenty-four hours, put the baby near a sunny window or take her outside for ten minutes once or twice daily, taking care to shield her eyes and avoid sunburn. As Susun Weed (1985) has commented, "Babies nearest to the window in hospitals are the least likely to become jaundiced."

When to cut the baby's umbilical cord after birth to best avoid jaundice has been a matter of disagreement between the medical and natural birth communities for many years. The argument for immediate cutting is that it prevents the blood in the placenta and cord from entering the baby's circulation, thus reducing the RBC load that the baby would otherwise have to convert or eliminate. But this method also reduces the amount of iron stores the baby could receive, possibly leading to an iron deficiency in the first year of life. In addition, the blood in the placenta and cord plays an important role in supporting the baby's cardiovascular system. Anne Frye (1990) recommends "not clamp[ing] the cord at birth. Wait until all pulsating has stopped at the navel base before cutting the cord (usually during the second hour of life). This gives the baby time to balance her bloodstream with the placenta and reduces jaundice." Delayed cutting also reduces the incidence of hemorrhage in the mother and the likelihood of another complication, retained placenta, which can also cause the mother to bleed excessively. (With twins the cord must be cut.)

Regardless of the baby's general health, most doctors recommend treatment on the basis of blood tests. Usually excessive, it includes exposing the baby to specialized lights and taking frequent blood samples for testing; it may be as extreme as a blood transfusion. All of these procedures carry physical risks and require separating the baby from the mother for the duration of the treatment.

If you and your health care provider determine that your baby's jaundice is physiological and you are treating the baby at home, your task is to support the baby's ability to clear out excess bilirubin. A healthy baby should have no trouble doing this. The following suggestions will help keep down the bilirubin level and resolve the jaundice:

- Nurse your baby frequently.
- Place the baby, as mentioned earlier, in indirect sunlight two to three times daily.
- Give the baby 3 to 5 drops of dandelion root tincture and 2 drops of alfalfa tincture four times daily.
- In severe cases, give the baby 1 to 2 droppers full of activated charcoal water every two hours. To prepare the solution, dilute 1 teaspoon of the charcoal powder in 1/4 cup of warm water. It can

be purchased at natural-food stores and some pharmacies, will temporarily turn the baby's poops black.

- The mother should drink 1 quart of Mother's Milk Tea I (see "Insufficient Milk Production" in Chapter 5) with catnip daily. In addition, she should take 30 to 50 drops of dandelion root tincture and 20 drops of alfalfa tincture three to four times a day, depending on the severity of the jaundice.

BREAST-MILK JAUNDICE

This form of jaundice is thought to be caused by a hormonal substance in the mother's milk that interferes with the breakdown of the baby's red blood cells. It usually develops around the fifth day after birth but can begin anywhere in the first couple of weeks. It can persist up to ten weeks. As long as your baby appears healthy, there is no cause for alarm. According to La Leche League, there is "no reason for even temporary weaning on this account."

If you feel that you must stop breast-feeding to let the bilirubin count decline, do so for no more than twenty-four to forty-eight hours. If you have a close friend or relative who is breast-feeding, you can let her nurse your baby or ask her to express some milk for your baby. (Note: AIDS can be passed through breast milk, so be careful of whom you let nurse your baby.) According to Anne Frye (1990), you can also give your baby goat's milk to which has been added 100 micrograms of folic acid per unfortified quart. During this time, express your own milk to prevent engorgement and maintain the flow. Remember, if your baby shows no signs of sickness or weakness, you need not suspend breast-feeding. In this case, use the herbal suggestions for physiological jaundice.

PATHOLOGICAL JAUNDICE

This form of jaundice is caused by a variety of internal problems in the baby, such as infection, blood incompatibility, and a damaged liver. Signs of pathological jaundice include jaundice that appears within the first forty-eight hours after birth and the symptoms of a sick baby described under "Physiological Jaundice." The baby is at risk of becoming anemic, dehydrated, and developing kernicterus. *Babies with pathological jaundice need to be treated by a physician.*

If you suspect that your baby needs medical care, seek it quickly. Regardless of treatment, you should insist upon remaining with your baby and maintaining your breast-feeding relationship. This is the best care the baby can receive. Do not underestimate the importance of your continued love and nourishment in ensuring your baby's optimal health.

❖ Vitamin K Shots ❖

Vitamin K is routinely given to newborns in the hospital, and parents often ask whether it is necessary for all babies. The reason it is used is that babies' blood-clotting mechanisms do not become fully established until the eighth day after birth; vitamin K is used to prevent hemorrhage in the newborn.

I do question whether this should be a routine practice. Nature's master plan gave babies low blood levels of vitamin K. In many years of attending births and conferring with midwives, I have never known a baby not receiving vitamin K to develop a hemorrhage after a normal birth. Hospital births have more potential for traumatic injury to occur, however. For example, the baby may be injured when forceps are used or during the cutting of the womb for a cesarean. The use of vitamin K in such circumstances may sometimes be warranted. Studies have shown that vitamin K given orally is equally as effective as that given by injection. If you choose to give your baby vitamin K, yet wish to spare your baby the pain of an injection, ask your practitioner to give the oral preparation.

Vitamin K is available to babies through the breast milk of their healthy mothers with no side effects. Injectable vitamin K carries the risk of side effects. To decrease the chance of vitamin K deficiency in your newborn, during the last six weeks of your pregnancy drink alfalfa and nettles tea. Place 1/4 ounce each of alfalfa and nettle leaves in a pint jar. Fill the jar with boiling water, steep for two hours, strain, and drink. The dosage is 2 cups a day. This is an excellent vitamin- and mineral-rich tea, noted to be specifically high in vitamin K as well as antihemorrhagic properties for mother and baby.

After the birth the mother can take 10 drops each of shepherd's purse and alfalfa tinctures two to three times a day, or can sip tea made with these herbs during the first few days of the postpartum.

Should your baby have significant bruising at the time of birth or any other injuries that may have resulted in internal bleeding, seek medical help promptly. A vitamin K injection or oral dose can be given at that time.

❖ Cradle Cap ❖

Cradle cap is an oily secretion from the baby's scalp that forms a crusty "cap" on the baby's head. (My six-year-old daughter lovingly and mistakenly calls it "baby crap.") It usually begins when the baby is about three months old and can persist until the child is two. It is not harmful, and regular hair washing (once or twice a week) with a mild shampoo will keep it to a minimum. In spots where it gets thick you can scratch it off as you shampoo.

- Rub the scalp with sesame, olive, or other vegetable oil. Then shampoo it off a few hours later.
- Wash the scalp with dilute Castile soap. This seems to "dry up" the secretion. Diluted witch hazel tea, rubbed into the scalp, is also an effective astringent.
- Place a handful of dry rolled oats into a small sock or cloth sack. Dampen the sack or sock and rub it well over the scalp while the oats become milky and lathery. This process will soften the cradle cap, which can then be removed with a fine-toothed comb.

❖ COLIC (OR THE "SUNSET BLUES") ❖

Colic is a catchall term for a condition in which a baby is fussy or uncomfortable despite being dry, warm, well fed, healthy, and loved. It may be caused by gas in the baby's intestines, or it may just be part of getting used to digestion and other bodily experiences. Colic is a difficult experience not only for the baby but also for the parents, who find it worrisome and exhausting. Some babies seem more prone to colic than others. Most outgrow it by four months.

Sometimes colic is just going to happen no matter what you do because your baby's digestive tract is just learning to work smoothly. Try to do your best to prevent it and to comfort your baby if it arises. Create calm and peaceful surroundings, but please don't blame yourself for your baby's discomfort. A couple of our kids always had a fussy time in the evening, so we began to jokingly refer to it as "the sunset blues." In fact, keeping a sense of humor was our most important remedy.

There is no foolproof method for preventing fussiness, but the following suggestions often help:

- Many babies get upset after their moms have eaten members of the cabbage family (broccoli, cabbage, kale, collards), turnips, garlic, onions, and spicy foods. Fried foods, peanuts, caffeine, dairy foods, eggs, beans, and wheat may also be aggravating.
- Hold your baby closely and firmly when you nurse, but don't fidget or distract the baby while he is eating, Nurse in quiet surroundings as often as possible. This will help to prevent indigestion.
- The following version of Mother's Milk Tea helps ease colic when taken by either mom or child and is also useful with hyperactivity, sleeplessness, and fussiness. A few teaspoons of this tea, unsweetened (honey is not safe for children under one year), can be

given directly to the baby. For more information about this tea, see "Insufficient Milk Production" in Chapter 5.

To prepare Mother's Milk Tea II, mix 1 ounce each of catnip leaves, chamomile flowers, and lemon balm leaves; 1/2 ounce of fennel seeds; and 1/4 ounce of lavender flowers. Store in a glass jar. Place 2 tablespoons of the mix in a cup of boiling water. Cover and steep for fifteen minutes. Strain, sweeten if desired, and drink while still warm. Breathe in the sweet, soothing scent as you drink.

- Dill, caraway, and anise seed teas are also useful for colic.
- If your baby has a regular fussy time, try to drink the tea before then. If possible, rest and eat well so you have the reserves you need to care for your baby without becoming exhausted and frazzled.
- Bach Rescue Remedy, a flower essence, is a well-used item in our fussy child repertoire. Give 2 drops to the baby and 4 drops each to mother and father.
- Massage and exercise the baby prior to the fussy period or at some point during it. Rub the baby's abdomen with warm hands and a bit of oil, using circular motions in a clockwise direction. Do this for fifteen minutes slowly and gently, talking or singing to your baby as you rub. Another massage technique is to rub gently in a downward motion from beneath the ribs to the lower abdomen, using the pinkie-finger side of your hands. Alternate your hands continually so it looks like you are making a water-wheel motion on your baby's belly.
- Exercise the baby's legs by "bicycling" them, together and alternately, up to the baby's abdomen. Press the legs up to the belly (both, then individually); then extend them back out and down. Do each motion five times slowly and smoothly.
- Put your baby in a baby sling and go for a walk. The closeness your baby will feel with you, combined with the rocking motions of your body, may soothe your baby and help her settle down. The outdoors has a soothing influence as well.

When followed by a warm bath, these techniques can be the basis of a pleasant ritual. With luck, the baby may even fall asleep. Remember, "this too shall pass." You won't always be able to take away your baby's suffering, but you can be there giving love and lending a soothing hand.

❖ THRUSH ❖

Thrush is another name for an infection of candida, or yeast. Candida is normally present in our bodies, but in certain circumstances it may get out of hand. In babies it produces a variety of discomforts, including red, irritated skin patches in the creases of the baby's neck, thighs, and armpits; white patches and sores in the mouth and on the tongue; a white pasty discharge in the folds of the vagina; and diaper rash. It can cause the baby to be irritable and gassy. If it spreads to the mother's nipples, it can make nursing very uncomfortable. Severe untreated thrush has the potential to turn into a major problem if the baby refuses to nurse or develops diarrhea. This is rare, however, and can be prevented by early recognition and treatment with natural home remedies.

If your nursing baby has thrush, be sure to treat your nipples with the remedies given below. For diaper rash associated with yeast, see "Baby's Skin Care and Rashes," earlier in this chapter.

A primary cause of thrush in a baby is use of antibiotics either directly or via the mother's breast milk. Antibiotics, while destroying unwanted organisms, also destroy the beneficial flora in the body that keep yeast and other organisms from proliferating. In their absence, a yeast infection can develop. A baby treated with antibiotics at birth is a prime candidate for thrush. Or a mother with a severe yeast infection can pass yeast onto the baby at birth. Yeast is also common in the environment, and any imbalance in the baby's system can allow this organism to proliferate.

GENERAL RECOMMENDATIONS

- Yeast thrives in dark, moist environments. Exposure to fresh air and sunlight is one of nature's best cures.
- For a thrush-related diaper rash, keep baby's bottom dry as much as possible. Let baby "air out" (nude, no diapers) each day.
- Nipple shields may contribute to yeast growth on your nipples. Don't wear them if thrush is a problem.
- Use excellent hygiene. Wash your hands after you change baby's diapers, touch your nipples, or touch the baby's mouth. This will prevent the thrush from spreading.

DIETARY RECOMMENDATIONS

- Drink plenty of water to ensure an abundant milk supply.
- Certain foods such as yeasted baked goods, wheat, sugars, honey, fruit and fruit juices, and heavy starches can contribute to yeast. Your diet should emphasize fresh vegetables, fish, beans, and whole grains such as rice and millet while you are treating the yeast infection. If the thrush clears up and then returns when you resume your regular diet, your baby is sensitive to something you are eating.

- Yogurt is one of the best home remedies for yeast infections. It helps restore a balance of organisms in the mouth and intestines. You can apply yogurt topically to inhibit yeast growth and soothe inflammation. Put a few spoonfuls of plain, unsweetened yogurt in a dish. If you apply the yogurt directly out of the container, you may contaminate the rest with yeast. Let the dish stand until the yogurt reaches room temperature. Using your fingers, a cotton swab, or a cotton ball, apply the yogurt liberally. For thrush in the baby's mouth, let the baby suck yogurt off of your (clean) fingers. Paint the insides of your baby's cheeks and his tongue with yogurt. Apply yogurt to your nipples and rinse them before each nursing.
- For yeast infections associated with antibiotics taken by the mother or baby, the mom should eat 2 to 3 tablespoons of plain, unsweetened yogurt with active cultures each day. The baby can be given 1 to 3 teaspoons of yogurt each day (in addition to that used above) by sucking it off your finger. The yogurt should always be at room temperature. Discontinue its use when the thrush or yeast rash has healed.
- You can use pure apple cider vinegar in place of the yogurt wash with equally good results, although the taste is less pleasant. If the baby is intolerant of dairy foods, this would be a good alternative. It is also the remedy of choice for washing mom's nipples. Dilute 1 tablespoon per 1/2 cup water.

Herbal Recommendations

- Dust slippery elm bark powder into the folds of the thighs and arms, under the neck, and on the fanny. It is soothing to irritated skin and helps absorb moisture. Wash the powder out of the creases and reapply a couple of times a day. In severe cases, add a pinch of goldenseal powder to each tablespoon of slippery elm to inhibit further yeast growth. Slippery elm makes a great baby powder and should replace commercial powders, which contain ingredients (like talc) known to be harmful to babies' respiratory systems and skin.
- Black walnut infusion or tincture can be painted in the baby's mouth and on the mother's nipples in tough cases. Apply two or three times a day. The mother can also take the tincture internally, 10 to 15 drops two to three times daily. Avoid getting it on clothing; it stains!

- A salve made with goldenseal, calendula, plantain, burdock, and chickweed will heal cracked and inflamed nipples. If necessary, suspend nursing on a particularly sore breast for twenty-four hours.

❖ TEETHING ❖

Baby teeth can come through the gums as early as the first few months after birth, but many babies don't have teeth until they are six to eight months old. Just as with walking and talking, the age when teeth first appear is an individual matter.

Likewise, babies display a variety of symptoms while teething, from none at all to great discomfort. While some pediatricians claim that teething does not cause cold symptoms, most parents will confirm that minor illness and fever often do accompany the eruption of teeth. Perhaps teething itself causes physical changes that manifest as symptoms of being unwell. Or it may be that the activity of teething temporarily increases susceptibility to illness.

Whatever the case may be, teething babies may correspondingly have fever, diarrhea, irritability, earache, runny noses, coughs, or general catarrh in the head or chest. (I recall that the eruption of my own wisdom teeth was accompanied by a nagging discomfort in my head and ears that bordered at times on pain.) While the baby may be "only teething," it is important not to disregard or minimize the attending discomforts because early attention to them can prevent them from becoming problems. This is an excellent time to provide herbs that not only soothe the child but also boost immunity and deal with infection if it is present.

A wealth of folk wisdom from many cultures demonstrates the ubiquitousness of teething problems. Here are some of the remedies common to Western herbalism. For suggestions regarding accompanying illnesses, see specific topics in this book.

Try any of these ideas singly or in combination to soothe a teething child:

- Give lots of love, comfort, and nursing.
- Mothers have relied on chamomile, lemon balm, and catnip for generations. They soothe a fussy baby's nerves and ease the pain. Mom can drink a brew of these herbs to keep calm and increase her patience as well. Since teething babies tend to wake more at night, this herbal mix is especially helpful because it can help mom and baby get a more restful sleep. The addition of a small amount of lavender is nice and adds to the restful qualities. Prepare

as a standard tea, using 1 tablespoon of the herbs in any combination to 1 cup of water; steep for fifteen minutes. For a very irritable baby (or mom!) increase the strength by steeping longer or using more herbs. This preparation can be taken safely in large amounts and over a long period of time. The baby can be given the tea by cup, spoon, or dropper, or by sucking a washcloth dipped in the tea. Of course, you can use a bottle, if you regularly use one anyway.

- Some find great benefit from homeopathic remedies. Hylands makes a good product called Homeopathic Teething Tablets. They are convenient to use and easily portable. Chamomila 30x is also considered a specific homeopathic for the general irritability associated with teething.

- Bach Rescue Remedy, a flower essence, is amazing for transforming a fretful, weepy baby into a restful, peaceful baby, and it works wonders for stressed parents, too. Give 4 drops of the "mother tincture" (the full-strength tincture) and repeat as needed, and rub some of the tincture straight onto the baby's gums for temporary pain relief.

- Although a strong-smelling herb, valerian tincture actually has a pleasant taste. It can be periodically given to babies and young children in dosages of 5 to 10 drops. It eases irritability; rubbed directly onto the gums, it also affords temporary pain relief. It is one of my favorite herbs for teething.

- Chickweed and burdock root are reliable for reducing gum inflammations. A tincture of these herbs in combination can be rubbed onto the gums. In fact, just gently rubbing the baby's gums at the site of the emerging tooth can be comforting.

- Brandy can be rubbed directly onto the baby's gums, or the baby can suck the corner of a washcloth that has been dipped in a bit of it. A very mild alcoholic beverage, it has been used traditionally for this purpose for centuries. I generally prefer not to use alcohol as a sedative if there are other remedies on hand, but if you are new to this and it's all you have at the moment, you can give it a try.

- Clove oil is another commonly known topical pain reliever for sore gums; however, it can be very irritating, even burning, so please try it on yourself before you use it on your baby. If you do use it, use only very small amounts.

PART III

NATURAL
HEALING
FOR CHILDREN

Chapter 8

❖

The Needs of
the Whole Child

Children are in a constant state of evolution and change that is nothing short of miraculous, flourishing with nourishment and conditions that meet their needs. To a great extent, the environment and circumstances in which children are raised influence how they grow and develop. As parents, we can have tremendous impact on the circumstances that help to shape and influence them. This chapter addresses some of the physical, emotional, intellectual, and spiritual needs of children and the ways in which we can provide the elements that sustain our children and foster their optimal unfolding.

❖ NUTURANCE ❖

Being well is not just eating the "right" foods or taking the "right" herbs. Emotional health and happiness are always important ingredients in the recipe for a healthy child. Even when your child is ill, the way in which you treat him or her creates long-lasting imprints of what caring is all about.

Nuturance does not mean "hothousing" kids (forcing them to grow unnaturally fast), overprotecting them or providing constant stimulation. Rather, it means taking the time to make children feel wanted and important, giving them love and understanding, with some encouragement sprinkled here and there, so they can unfold gracefully at their own pace. They need someone to truly take an interest in them, to listen to them with the intention of hearing who they are, even if they are being loud, wild, or independent minded (often referred to as "disobedient"). Children need to be patiently listened to and answered thoughtfully.

Nurturance is also the act of cultivating in children, by example, humanitarian values through prosocial behavior—that is, how to be caring, considerate, and empathetic people. Health can only truly exist if we are working toward the health of our whole human family. Otherwise, we are only dealing with the health of the body, not the whole person.

Home health care is an ideal way to teach children these positive values. By seeing and engaging in health-promoting behaviors in their daily lives, children come to model them. And the best way for them to learn is through our example.

❖ WARMTH ❖

That warmth is a basic human survival need seems obvious, but the need for warmth on a daily basis as a contributor to optimal growth and development is frequently overlooked. Digestion and assimilation depend on warmth in our bodies. These days people are accustomed to artificial heating and cooling, so there seems little need to dress appropriately for the seasons—we can go to and from air-conditioned cars and buildings without considering how extreme temperature changes affect us, eat foods right out of the fridge, drink and eat summer foods in the winter. These habits can wreak havoc in our bodies as they are already doing to the Earth. I have seen that when children regularly consume cold foods and drinks in the cold months, they are much more prone to coughs and colds, earaches and runny noses. Our relationship to warmth is very basic to our lack of harmony with nature. To regain this harmony, we don't have to be rigidly inflexible and never have ice cream or iced tea. Rather, it is a practical matter of listening to nature. When it's cold, we need to be warm; when it's hot, we need to be cool but not freeze ourselves.

We can also teach our children (as we learn!) to dress appropriately for the time of year and day just as animals shed and grow fur with the seasons. We can protect our inner heat in the winter by wearing hats and keeping the chest and abdomen warm. Little girls who wear dresses in winter should have adequate protection for their legs and genitals as they can be more prone to urinary tract infections from exposure to drafts. We can also prevent earaches by teaching children to keep their heads covered. These simple measures go a long way in preventing illness.

In human terms, warmth is more than a temperature measurable on a thermometer. We also use the word to refer to a tangible quality of human love. It is what babies and children (and adults, too) long to be enveloped in. It is the essence of life that incubates growth. From this spiritual warmth children gain an unseen force for growth without which their lives would be bleak. Studies have confirmed that babies and children left in isolation without human warmth exhibit failure to thrive. Warmth is a welcoming feeling that says, "You are wanted here; you are loved." Without it, health cannot long be maintained. And that brings us back full circle to our need for nurturance.

❖ Rhythms ❖

Babies gestate to the sounds of the placenta, their mothers' heartbeats, and their own heartbeats. The rhythms of these sounds fluctuate according to the mother's moods and activities, but for the most part they are pretty regular. The child depends upon these rhythms as part of his sense of security. Research has shown that playing a tape recording of gestational sounds, particularly the mother's heartbeat, has a calming influence on infants, and that premature babies exposed to maternal heart sounds show faster developmental rates than preemies who are not exposed to these sounds, even though they receive the same level of medical care.

A healthy child establishes her own breathing patterns almost immediately after birth. The rhythm of inhalation and exhalation, as well as the heartbeat, accompanies us constantly for the entirety of our lives. Humans live by cycles known as "circadian rhythms." The natural world has its own rhythms as well: The sun rises and sets, the moon waxes and wanes, the seasons change, the tides change. Beings in harmony with nature live by a rhythm—an inner clockwork if you will—that keeps them in harmony with the greater movements of the planet.

Those of us who live in cities and modernized environments are usually unaware of natural rhythms. We eat and sleep at all hours, have light whenever we wish via electricity, and regulate the temperatures in our homes. Our schedules of work and schooling are often incongruent with our human needs, demanding of us that we be in certain places at certain times regardless of whether we have had the chance to eat or use the bathroom, for example. This is very different from the days when we went to sleep when it was dark, ate foods according to their seasonal availability, and lived lives that reflected, rather than defied, natural rhythms.

Providing children from a young age with regularity in their lives and exposure to natural cycles gives them a sense of natural rhythms and timing. An abundance of outdoor experiences so that they can learn for themselves the smell of rain, the feeling of atmospheric pressure before a thunderstorm, and the phases of the moon; so that they can awaken with the sun and sleep with the moon; so that they have quiet times to explore their own inner landscapes—all contribute to this awareness.

Rhythms are not rigid or static but flowing processes. It takes commitment and persistence on the part of adults to create for their children a rhythmic environment in the midst of busy, hectic, and, at times, chaotic lifestyles. When the life around them is rhythmic, children are able to keep their own rhythms, which helps in the proper functioning of their bodies and therefore is essential in preventing illness. An additional benefit may be an appreciation for the world that surrounds them and a sense of responsibility for the environment.

As natural imitators seeking to gather information about how to be in the world, children emulate not only what we do but also how we do it. Here's an example of this idea that I once read: A child was watching a man hammering nails. The man was obviously angry, possibly about an incident that had occurred earlier that day. The child, seeking to fully embody the actions of the adult, began to hammer just like the adult— angrily! Since emotions are so closely related to our heart and respiratory rates and thus our overall physiological processes, both what we do and how we do it influences our children's ability to function smoothly. When we frequently treat children in ways that cause them anger, hurt, dejection, or insecurity, we alter their inner rhythms in ways that promote illness, not health. Of course, no parent is perfect, kind, and gentle all the time. Parents argue; life has its ups and downs. Intense emotions such as anger, sadness, and frustration are as much a part of life as love, but in considering ways to promote well-being in children, we cannot overlook how what we are modeling influences them.

Perhaps the best way to practice proper modeling is to learn to manage our own anger. Too often we let anger or frustration about work, money, relationships, or other matters spill into our interactions with our kids. Not having an adult perspective, they may not empathize with our feelings and may internalize our responses to them, leading to a deep sense of anxiety. By practicing relaxation techniques, talking over our problems with an understanding friend, or even practicing expressive therapies to help us discharge our own tensions and anger appropriately and productively, we provide healthy modeling for our children.

❖ PLAY AND NATURAL ELEMENTS ❖

Earth, water, fire, air—these are the elements that make up our world. Children love to explore piles of earth, play with buckets of mud, in puddles of rain, and on swings, fly kites, climb trees. It is healthy and appropriate for children to get dirty! Let's not teach them that "dirt"— Earth—is bad. Let's encourage their explorations—just put them in old clothes and let 'em go. Our attitudes influence their perceptions. We can teach them that a puddle of fresh rainwater is unpleasantly wet and cold or that playing in it can be fun. Unless they are ill, let them be filled with play in the elements. Pure outdoor play followed by a warm bath and a cup of tea with homemade cookies make an afternoon to nourish body and soul. I assure you that your child will sleep well that night.

Most children also relish the opportunity to explore fire—bonfires, candles, matches. We can teach our children about the life-sustaining qualities of heat and fire by teaching them to safely strike matches, light candles, and start fires in the woodstove, fireplace, or campground. Young children will gain a sense of confidence by accomplishing these "dangerous" tasks, and given such a privilege, they will learn to respect safety rules. Their sense of importance and competence supports their self-esteem, and thus their health, in deep and lasting ways.

As we offer opportunities for our children to explore, we can enhance their imagination by providing them with tools and toys made primarily of natural materials. These may include wood for building, sandboxes, watering cans, shovels, and pots for playing outdoors; dolls made of natural fibers and toys of wood and cloth for indoors. Natural materials have more of a feeling of life and character than toys made of plastic, which is derived from petroleum. Often, plastic toys are firmly fixed into certain gestures, allowing little room for transformation. Playthings that can be many sorts of things encourage creativity. With a few basic materials children can create a palace. Of course, a commitment to using materials that are environmentally friendly also gives kids a familiarity from a young age with the idea of making choices that are environmentally conscious.

How much television our children watch also requires some critical attention. Most view television for many hours each day. Aside from the possible harmful effects of radiation emissions, the very act of watching TV may also be harmful. Images on the screen appear in such rapid succession that a child barely has time to integrate one image before another appears. And the content of the images and programming is frequently insulting or frightening to children's sensibilities. Violence and sexuality, for example, are common themes that may be presented before children are emotionally ready to deal with these topics, creating confusion, tension, and even nightmares. Such themes may be reenacted on playgrounds as children attempt to understand and emulate what they are seeing. Unfortunately, violence and early sexuality among teenagers may be, in part, a reflection of the images that they have internalized through television viewing.

If we want our children to be healthy, we must make every effort to provide healthful images for them to emulate and positive ideas for them to incorporate into their lives. Not all television watching is inherently bad, but activities that teach kids real-life skills or crafts or even just time playing outdoors are preferable to sitting idly being passively entertained. Kids and parents together can plant gardens (even in the inner cities), visit parks, draw, cook, or do something nice for a neighbor. As we improve the quality of our immediate environment, we can influence the environment all around us.

❖ FREEDOM AND GUIDANCE ❖

We are conditioned to seeing children as immature adults, incapable of independent thought and action, and yet they have a great capacity for making wise decisions. Trusting children is an art. Learning to listen to them and allowing them to make choices for themselves, while still giving them the guidance that helps them feel secure and keeps them safe, takes time and is an ever-evolving process because their needs, boundaries, and areas of exploration continue to change and grow. One day they are learning to walk down steps; the next day they are learning to drive the car. We have to rely on our inner guidance and on good communication with our kids to guide us through the rough spots.

Knowing when to insist upon something and when to let go always takes thought, and clearly there are times for each. For example, it is wise to insist that a child wear a warm hat on a cold, windy day, but if left to their own resources most kids are sensible enough to come to the same conclusion. But insisting that a child eat even though she doesn't want to may not be wise, unless, of course, she has health problems that are causing a poor appetite and she is losing weight. Maintaining a light diet for a few days is an excellent way to prevent or lessen the severity of an oncoming cold. Many times children instinctively know they should skip a meal or even fast for a day though they may not be able to explain their behavior. On the other hand, recent studies on obesity suggest that forcing children to eat meals, after expressing that they've had enough food, causes children to ignore the body's message of fullness. Done repeatedly, it may lead to a shutting down of this innate, self-regulatory mechanism, resulting in people who become overweight because they don't know when to stop eating.

So many times we say "No, No, No" when saying "Yes" is harmless and very easy. We too often resent cleaning up messes made as children learn new skills, such as fixing their own snacks, and so we replace their desire to learn, explore, and grow with fear of disapproval. We end up with kids who either stop trying to do new and challenging tasks or continue to explore but do it behind our backs. Taking this time out of our already busy schedules to enjoy the world with our children may seem like a burden, but if you do so, you will be reawakened to treasures, adventures, and splendors you have long forgotten or perhaps never known.

Finding the balance between guidance and freedom seems to lie in the art of listening to the message of our children's actions—looking at our kids from a broad perspective and with parental concern, not parental anxiety. The most important thing about guidance is not to let it become a control issue or power struggle with our kids. When we express reasonable concerns to our children, respecting that they are intelligent human beings who want to be in good relationship with us, they will hear what we are saying. Children need both guidance and freedom for physical and emotional health. Children need freedom to stretch their limbs and exercise their wills, with enough of a boundary to know that we are with them and will not let them down in an ocean of choices and wide open space. Always ask yourself if a limit or boundary is reasonable and necessary before you impose it. If it's not, your child will feel that you are just being controlling, and this will hinder an open relationship between you. Our kids can be our greatest allies if we don't alienate them but learn to enlist their trust and cooperative (not compliant) spirits.

❖ SECURITY ❖

This world can be pretty scary. From wars on foreign soils and crossfire from drug wars in housing projects and neighborhoods, to child molesters in schools and day care centers, our children grow up in a world with many dangers. As parents we have the formidable responsibility of preparing them to face the realities of life, which at some point, often all too early, they must understand for their safety.

Children expect our honesty, and, in fact, they cannot be shielded from everything. But we can buffer them so they don't take on more than necessary. Children are sensitive on a psychic level, as we all once were and still can be. They don't need all the problems of the world spelled out to them, and they don't need to feel insecurity and fear. Saint George—a favorite fairy-tale character of many children—used his shield to protect himself from the dragon until he was ready to emerge from behind it and deliver the fatal blow. We can—and should—provide shielding to our children until they are ready and able to step beyond our protection.

At some point—this is different for each child but often takes place around age nine—a child becomes capable of an intellectual understanding of the world's problems and dangers, which although still frightening, won't paralyze him or her with the irrational fears that a very young child might experience. For example, a friend recently told me that her young son heard that an adult friend of theirs had been fired from his job. The child, visibly disturbed by this information, asked if his dad would be fired as well. Upon further discussion with her son, the mother discovered that he thought being "fired" meant being burned.

Protection or shielding does not mean that we should forbid children to climb trees or jungle gyms or take other calculated risks that are a normal part of childhood. Children need to be able to have a lot of fun! It just means that we keep what enters their awareness as non-threatening as possible. Children are entitled to a childhood, and it is a gift we can allow them to have.

Everyone is entitled to go to sleep and wake up feeling safe, yet many people all over the world face terrible conditions in their daily lives. So while shielding our children from issues that they are yet unable to comprehend, we ought not teach them to be inconsiderate of the pain and suffering of others. If we can help them mature into caring and compassionate adults—for example, by assisting in the home care of siblings who are ill, tending gardens, caring for pets, or even helping in a homeless shelter or home for the aged—we can encourage a generation of people to work toward reducing suffering in our world.

While we cannot prevent inevitable illness, or meet our children's every need, we can recognize that our kids are unique individuals with complex emotions. Looking at the needs of the whole child can enable us to provide them with the elements they require for wellness, address the root of a problem should one arise, and prevent it from recurring. Rather than putting a topical solution on a problem that may be more than skin deep, true health care penetrates to the needs of the soul.

Chapter 9

❖

Natural Remedies for Children's Complaints: An A–Z Guide

No matter how prepared or knowledgeable you are, a sick child is likely to be upsetting, even if just to the routines of your home and family life. To some degree this is how it should be, because illness tends to make us slow down, take stock of what is going on with the person who is sick, and evaluate what may have brought it about.

As you develop your powers of observation and intuition, you will begin to recognize early and subtle signs from your child that he or she is coming on to an illness. See "Common Early Signs of Illness" in Chapter 3 for more on this topic.

I've seen two main categories of illnesses in children. One is what I call "growth spurt illness"; the other is sickness. You can often recognize the source of your child's illness by taking a heartfelt look at what's been going on in your child's life and at his or her age.

This is especially true with the growth-spurt type of illness. I have seen many children get "sick," especially with fevers, just before making a big developmental step—such as walking, speaking new words, cutting teeth, and doing other new things. It's as if they need to let go of their bodies just a little, only to evolve a little more fully when the illness passes.

Children also become sick as a direct result of stress and overstimulation. A clear example of this happened with my first child. When he was about two and a half years old, my husband and I had an argument next to his bed while he was sleeping. We were literally over his head—my husband was on one side of him near one ear, and I was on the other side right next to his other ear. It wasn't such a loud argument, but we were expressing a lot of anger. Well, at five o'clock the next morning, our son woke up screaming and writhing around, with—you guessed it—an ear inflammation, his first and only bout with this common childhood occurrence. This really taught us a lesson about the subtle energies that support health and encourage illness. He recovered within a few hours with the excellent help of herbs and massage—and a lot of apologies and love between all of us—but the experience left a strong impression on me. Some may dismiss the event as merely coincidental, but other parents have confirmed it with their own experiences. Moreover, in recent years, many medical practitioners have begun to recognize the correlation between stress and the onset of illness.

Illness serves as a stimulus to our children's immune systems, causing them to mature and to develop resistance (immunity) to many of the organisms in their environment. Just as we strengthen our characters by going through challenges that bring out our full human potential, our children develop their immune systems by using them. In fact, developing immunities seems to be the purpose of many childhood illnesses, which are usually harmless, unless they occur in adulthood, when they may be of greater consequence. These illnesses enable us to develop in and evolve with our environment.

Natural healing is founded on the belief that our bodies are designed to maintain well-being. The remedies natural health care practitioners use *assist* the body's healthy response to illness. We attempt to support and nurture, not suppress and kill organisms without addressing the source of the problem.

Before getting into specific complaints and remedies, I want to say a bit about guilt. When we talk about preventing illness, we necessarily talk about what actions may lead to illness. But there are times, even with the most healthy lifestyle, when aches, pains, and sickness will occur. If we think we can conquer or escape illness by living "purely and cleanly," we are creating the inner stress of always fighting or trying to avoid something. This creates an enormous amount of performance pressure and limitation in experiencing life, as well as disappointment, frustration, and shame when illness inevitably arises.

Health is not just the absence of illness, it is also the flexibility to deal with the unexpected challenges that life may present us, including illnesses. By attending to illness in others with grace and hope, we model compassion to our children. As we learn to accept our own illnesses (and other imperfections) we give ourselves unconditional love. This is the basis from which true healing arises, and it is a gift worth passing on to our children.

Included below you will find descriptions of the most common complaints and illnesses that are likely to occur in children and a variety of natural remedies for them, including herbs, dietary suggestions, massage and other external techniques, and practical wisdom. These remedies have shown themselves to be consistently effective, are safe when used correctly, and require only generally accessible supplies. In addition, information is provided on when to seek medical care.

The remedies included in this chapter may be used quite success-fully by adults although frequently in larger doses. Many of the internal remedies are not suitable for pregnant women, however. I have tried to note these, but if you are pregnant, please consult with an experienced herbalist or refer to books specifically on pregnancy wellness before tak-ing any internal remedies.

❖ ABSCESSES ❖

Abscesses are localized sacs or pockets of infection that may drain or ooze pus. Red and inflamed in appearance, they are very painful and may cause a fever. Mild local infections that go untreated for many days often become abscessed. Areas that sustain repeated damage or irrita-tion can also become abscessed (for example, a stubbed or scraped toe rubbing inside a snug shoe). Gums and teeth can abscess as a result of a local irritation (such as a popcorn hull stuck between the teeth and gums), an injury, or tooth decay. Abscesses can be treated at home, except for those caused by tooth decay, in which case you will need to get dental attention. An embedded foreign object causing inflammation and pain will need to be removed. This can usually be done with water and perhaps a gently applied toothbrush or toothpick.

Healing an abscess requires diligent attention and consistent effort. You will usually be rewarded with quick and complete recovery. Some improvement should be noticeable within twenty-four hours. Usually the inflammation gets concentrated and pus comes to the surface and drains, or the infection is reabsorbed, resolving itself. You can *gently* massage the area to facilitate this process. When the pus begins to clear, the inflammation subsides along with the pain, which is caused by the pressure of the pus under the skin.

WHEN TO SEEK MEDICAL CARE

Unresponsive abscesses can become serious systemic infections. Watch your child carefully. Any worsening of the child's general health, including an increase in temperature, may indicate that the infection is spreading. Red streaks emanating from the site of the abscess indicate blood poisoning. If you notice either of these changes, you need to seek further help. Blood poisoning can *quickly* become life threatening, and antibiotics will be necessary.

General Recommendations

The treatment of abscesses requires a combination of internal and external remedies. The internal remedies and dietary suggestions are the same regardless of the abscess's location, although external applications for skin and oral abscesses vary. After familiarizing yourself with the necessary internal remedies, refer to the appropriate external treatments that follow. In all cases, make sure your child gets extra rest.

Dietary Recommendations

- Probably the most important remedy for any infection is to drink a lot of water. Half a cup per hour is an adequate amount for younger children (up to seven years), more as age and body size increase. You are trying to flush the system, cool the abscess's internal heat, and keep the child well hydrated.
- Provide a light diet consisting of fresh fruits, vegetables, and whole grains. Avoid dairy foods, flour products, meats, and rich and processed foods. At least 1 cup daily of freshly made apple, carrot, or beet juice, alone or in combination, is particularly beneficial. These juices nourish the lymphatic system and encourage the blood to eliminate infections.
- In addition, give the child 500 milligrams of vitamin C four times a day.

Herbal Recommendations

- Every two to four hours, depending on the severity of the infection, orally administer echinacea tincture (1 drop for every 2 pounds of body weight). Along with this, give 10 drops each of fresh plantain, chickweed, and burdock root tinctures, or alternatively, an infusion of these herbs in equal parts. They are excellent for assisting the immune system in clearing the infection and "cooling" the heat that accompanies it; in addition, the infection is less likely to spread as you work with the external remedies to heal the abscess.
- Drinking plentiful quantities of chickweed tea is helpful (add a pinch of salt for a delicious broth). Chickweed is a common and abundant weed worth the effort of learning to identify in your neighborhood. Consult a field guide or botanist for identification.
- For severe abscesses, add goldenseal tincture to the above formula (1 drop per 5 pounds of body weight). After the infection has disappeared, give the child 2 tablespoons of unsweetened yogurt daily to restore intestinal flora that may have been upset by goldenseal's antibiotic properties.

- Continue the internal remedies (with the exception of goldenseal) for twenty-four hours after the infection is clearly gone.

EXTERNAL REMEDIES FOR SKIN ABSCESSES

Skin abscesses may occur anywhere on the body but are common on fingers and toes because they are susceptible to getting stubbed, stepped on, or smashed.

- Moist heat is critically important. Soak the area in water as hot as can be tolerated (taking care to avoid burning) three times a day for twenty minutes each time. If possible add 1 teaspoon calendula tincture and 1/4 cup Epsom salts per quart of water.
- After each soak, apply the following poultice. Place in a dish and mix enough macerated (chopped and mashed) fresh plantain leaves to cover the area (chickweed can be substituted); goldenseal, echinacea, and chaparral powders in equal parts (1/2 teaspoon of the mix per plantain leaf); green clay (1 teaspoon per plantain leaf); and enough water to make a paste.

  Smear the poultice well on the affected part, cover with a clean gauze or cloth, and then place a hot-water bottle or heating pad on the area. Change the dressing each time you soak the abscess. Try to continually keep moist heat on the area until the infection subsides.

REMEDIES FOR TOOTH AND GUM ABSCESSES

- Rinse the mouth at least three times daily with 1/4 cup warm water to which has been added 1/2 teaspoon sea salt and 1/4 teaspoon myrrh powder.
- Squeeze 10 to 15 drops combined of echinacea root, burdock root, and dandelion root tinctures directly onto the inflammation every two to four hours. This will bring almost immediate pain relief. You can use a strong decoction of these same herbs as a rinse if the tinctures are unavailable. Repeat as often as needed.
- When you make chickweed tea as suggested earlier, save the plant material and use it as a poultice on the affected spot. Remove the poultice when it becomes warm and replace it with a fresh one.
- Have the child sleep or rest on a hot-water bottle to relieve tension in the affected area and promote healthy circulation. This facilitates the body's natural response. Inflammation itself results in of the extra circulation of blood, which combats and digests the infection; pus is the shedding of the white blood cells eating the bacteria that have invaded the damaged or irritated tissue.

❖ Aches ❖

Like adults, children can experience occasional aches and sore muscles, particularly after participating in sports or other strenuous activities. In addition, children often feel achy and irritable when ill or feverish.

- For general aches, chamomile, lemon balm, and catnip teas, alone or in combination, will bring steady relief. Valerian tincture, 1 drop per 5 pounds of body weight, is also soothing to a fretful, achy child.
- A massage with oil that contains chamomile, lavender, or St. John's wort, or an herbal bath made with any of these in the form of infusions or oils, also eases sore muscles or heavy spirits.
- For specific sore areas or muscles, rub arnica oil or a warming liniment that contains herbs or oils such as cinnamon, wintergreen, or camphor directly onto the area. Dit Dat Jiao, an excellent Chinese herbal liniment, can sometimes be found in shops that sell Chinese herbal products.
- Warm up a pillow stuffed with chamomile blossoms by tossing it in the dryer for a few minutes. Applying it directly to the aches or sleeping on it provides comfort.
- For children who are achy during a fever, use these suggestions in conjunction with remedies for fevers.

❖ Acne ❖

The skin is a major organ of elimination: What goes in the body comes out via the skin. Foods high in nutrients and low in chemical additives, heavy oils, and hard-to-digest starches decrease the likelihood of developing acne. If skin problems are already apparent, they will clear up more quickly with dietary improvements. Herb foods such as burdock root, dandelion greens, nettles, chickweed, red clover, shiitake mushrooms, and green vegetables and seaweed eaten as a regular part of the diet will also help prevent skin problems.

Hygiene is also important to the skin's health. Teach children to keep themselves clean by washing daily with warm water and a wash cloth. A gentle, mild, Castille, glycerine, or olive oil-based soap may be used. Daily washing helps clean both the substances coming from within the body as well as those coming from the air and is especially important in big cities, where we are constantly exposed to air laden with dust and pollutants.

Teenagers may develop acne because of increasing hormone levels, stress, lack of adequate sleep, and a tendency toward eating fast foods.

Even kids raised on natural foods may experiment with their diets and develop acne. Girls may be particularly prone to acne before their periods begin each month.

DIETARY RECOMMENDATIONS

- Discourage your child from eating chocolate, fatty meats, sugar, fried foods, oily nuts (peanuts and cashews, for example), cheese, butter, and ice cream for the duration of the outbreak.
- Emphasize a diet rich in fresh vegetables and fruits, whole grains, and beans, supplemented by fresh chicken or fish (preferably organic).
- Healthy elimination will lessen the burden of elimination via the skin. Teach children excellent eating and elimination habits when they are young, and teenage and adult acne will not become a significant problem.
- If constipation occurs, it must be attended to. See "Constipation" for remedies.

HERBAL RECOMMENDATIONS

- Combine 2 ounces each of dried burdock root and nettle leaves and 1 ounce each of chickweed, red clover blossoms, sarsaparilla, and dandelion root. Prepare an infusion using 1 ounce of herbs to 1 quart water. Dosage is 2 cups daily. The tea may be used for an extended period of time; stop the treatment for five days after each month on the tea.
- Echinacea root is an excellent internal remedy for skin infections and persistent acne. Use 1 drop per 5 pounds of body weight (for example, someone weighing 120 pounds should take 24 drops) three or four times a day. *Or* add 1 ounce of the dried roots of *Echinacea angustifolia* to the above infusion.
- Herbal steam directed toward the face or affected parts can open and cleanse the pores. This is done by leaning (carefully) over a pot of very hot, steaming water or, preferably, a hot infusion of burdock root or calendula blossoms for about ten minutes. A towel draped over the head and the pot will help direct the steam to the face.
- Alternatively, place a *hot* (but not burning) compress of calendula blossoms, burdock root, or chickweed infusion on the affected areas. Whether you use steam or an infusion, thoroughly wash the face afterward with a cloth and a pure, mild soap that contains no chemical additives or heavy perfumes. Follow this by splashing the area with distilled witch hazel or cool with witch hazel infusion (1/4 ounce to 1 pint water).

The herbs used for the facial steam and compress are cleansing and antimicrobial. They also reduce inflammation. The heat dilates the pores of the skin, which are then washed free of oils and secretions. Witch hazel is an astringent that helps reduce the volume of the secretions as well as closes the pores.

- For deep or mildly infected pimples, use a hot compress as described. Then apply a dab of honey or a thin paste of green clay to the pimple and allow to dry. Apply twice a day. These will draw the pimple to the surface.

❖ Anemia (Iron Deficiency) ❖

Iron is a mineral that our entire body requires for healthy, rich blood, adequate oxygenation, and proper immune-system health. A deficiency of this mineral, called "anemia," may occur in children whose diets are incomplete or whose absorption of iron is inefficient. Common signs of anemia are pale complexion, fatigue, chilliness or cold hands and feet, finicky eating, shortness of breath, and sometimes repeated infections or colds.

Including daily servings of iron-rich foods and herbs can help your child (or you) build healthy blood. However, one needn't be anemic to enrich his or her diet with any of the following blood builders.

Dietary Recommendations

- Foods that are iron-rich include raisins, prunes, dried apricots, dried cherries, currants, black mission figs, leafy green vegetables such as kale and collard greens, beets, beans, molasses, red meat, seaweed, and spirulina. You'll be amazed how readily some kids will eat prunes soaked or stewed in apple juice, "candied" corn (popcorn coated with warm molasses and honey, then baked) and kidney bean burritos. Get your kids to brush their teeth after eating dried fruits to prevent cavities.
- Vitamin C enhances iron absorption and caffeinated foods (such as chocolate) lower it. Give your child 250 milligrams of vitamin C or a fruit or vegetable rich in C along with iron-rich foods. An excellent supplement would be to give your child 1 tablespoon of blackstrap molasses along with the vitamin C twice daily.
- Drinking milk can inhibit iron absorption, so let your child have milk separately from iron-rich foods.
- Kelp powder and dulse flakes are dried sea vegetables that may be sprinkled directly onto foods. A teaspoon to a tablespoon of kelp powder daily or a few tablespoons of dulse flakes daily is a healthy iron and calcium supplement. Taste for the foods is acquired, but

many kids really enjoy them. Dulse can be toasted in the oven or a skillet for a few minutes and then eaten like chips for a snack. It can also be sprinkled onto oatmeal and popcorn or cooked into soups. Kelp is also available in whole, dried form (called "Kombu"), which can be cut into small pieces or left in a strip about 6 inches long and cooked into stews, soups, or beans. The Kombu can be eaten with the dish or discarded.

Herbal Recommendations

- *Nettles:* Make an infusion by steeping a handful of the dried herb in 1 quart boiling water. Steep for two hours. Let the child drink a cup of this every day. You can be sweeten it with honey or apple juice, add it to soups, or flavor it with a "bouillon" cube.
- *Iron tonic syrup:* In ancient times, herbs were used as foods as well as remedially and as seasoning. Unfortunately, modern diets have become increasingly limited and generally exclude many of the plants our ancestors consumed. Used as foods even in small supplementary amounts, herbs can supply us with a variety of easily assimilable nutrients, some of which may be missing from the foods we buy at the market.

  Commercial iron supplements are frequently hard to digest and can cause constipation. This iron tonic is easy to digest and is even a gentle, natural laxative. It also provides other trace minerals, strengthens the liver and digestive system, and enhances the body's overall assimilation of nutrients.

  To prepare, steep 1/2 ounce each of dried yellow dock and dandelion roots in 1 pint boiling water. Cover the container while steeping, and let sit for four to eight hours. Strain the liquid into a small pot and reduce by simmering to 3/4 cup of liquid. Add 1/4 cup honey or a combination of honey and molasses (molasses increases the iron value). Let cool to room temperature and store in a bottle in the refrigerator. The tonic keeps for up to three months.

  Iron tonic syrup is for children two years and older. The dosage is 1 to 3 teaspoons daily for children, 1 to 2 tablespoons daily for teenagers and adults.
- Other herbs considered to enhance iron levels are alfalfa, burdock root, parsley, and chickweed.

❖ Appetite Loss ❖

All children go through cycles in their eating habits. Sometimes they eat more, and sometimes they eat less. Children eat intuitively. They usually won't eat when not hungry, tired, or sick, and they may prefer to eat frequent small snacks rather than three "solid" meals a day. Children may also have preferences about how foods are prepared and served. For example, they may not like their foods mixed together, or they may prefer raw carrots to steamed carrots. While it is best not to overindulge picky habits, there is nothing wrong with providing favorite foods as long as they are healthful. Enjoyment of food is important to good appetite.

A child who generally eats well and then suddenly begins to skip meals may be said to have appetite loss. This may also be the case with a child who is usually a finicky eater. When a child suddenly loses appetite, he or she may be getting a cold. Trusting their intuitive resistance to eating may be best. Offer tea, broth, warm apple juice, and plenty of water. Once the cold has passed, a healthy appetite will return. Don't, however, *force* a sick child to fast; just provide simple foods. When we are sick, our bodies require nutrients to heal and recover.

Sweet foods, large snacks, and even too many liquids close to meals dampen appetite. Hunger is probably the finest appetite stimulant known. If your child needs snacks, try to provide them well in advance of meals, or provide a light snack of vegetable sticks and maybe a healthful dip if the child is hungry and the meal is not quite ready.

Emotional stress can interfere with a child's appetite. If you suspect this, try to understand and help your child resolve the problem. Children are sensitive to disharmony at home and in school. Both Mother's Milk Tea II (see "Colic [or the Sunset Blues]" in Chapter 7) and Calm Child Formula (see "Car Sickness" in this chapter) are especially suited to soothing kids under stress. Seek supportive counseling if necessary.

Anemia (iron deficiency) or intestinal parasites can lead to a chronically poor appetite. If you suspect either of these, refer to the appropriate sections in this book for further information.

WHEN TO SEEK MEDICAL CARE

For prolonged lack of appetite accompanied by weight loss, seek a physician's help. Don't overlook the possibility of anorexia or bulimia in older children and teenagers.

HERBAL RECOMMENDATIONS

- Aromatic herbs such as fennel, anise, dill, coriander, cardamom, and caraway seeds stimulate the appetite. Make a tea by pouring boiling water over 1 tablespoon of any of these seeds, cover immediately, and steep for ten minutes. Sweeten with 1/2 teaspoon honey or apple juice if desired. Serve one hour before meals if possible. You should notice some improvement within a week of using these herbs regularly.

- Dandelion root and agrimony are both stomach and digestive tonics that stimulate the appetite. In fact, most herbs sold as "bitters" serve this function. You can give your child 10 to 15 drops of both of these tinctures two to three times daily to promote a healthy appetite.
- As often as possible, offer foods that are flavorful, mildly spicy, or otherwise appealing to your child until she regains her appetite. Bland food is *not* an appetite enhancer!

❖ ASTHMA ❖

The feeling of not being able to breathe is extremely frightening. A person with asthma has attacks of difficult breathing, wheezing, and sometimes other symptoms such as tiredness (from lack of oxygen), chest pain, loss of appetite, and watery, itchy eyes. Attacks may last for a few hours or a few days. Asthma usually begins in childhood, and although it can persist into adulthood, it is commonly outgrown.

Allergies can trigger asthma attacks. Avoiding foods that are common allergens (eggs, dairy products, peanut butter, chocolate, corn, wheat, artificial additives) as well as environmental pollutants (dust, cigarette smoke, pollen, animal hair, woolen garments, carpeting, fumes) can reduce the incidence of attacks.

Some consider asthma to be a stress-related illness. Divorce or difficulty in the parental relationship or a death in the family can cause enormous stress in a child. The idea that our children's illnesses can be related to stress in the home or in school is not meant to lay blame on or cause guilt in parents. Rather, we need to be aware that children are perceptive of our troubles and sometimes have troubles of their own. Since children commonly internalize problems, any child going through a crisis needs extra support.

Colds and respiratory infections can lead to asthma attacks in a child with this condition, so try to catch them early. Excitement and exertion can also be triggers. Asthmatic children should not be considered or feel debilitated by their condition; however, care does need to be taken to prevent attacks.

WHEN TO SEEK MEDICAL CARE

Severe asthma attacks can be life threatening. If your child is at all unable to catch his or her breath or has any blueness of the skin, seek medical help immediately! Seek help promptly if mild symptoms persist despite the use of natural remedies. In both mild and severe cases your child needs your calming reassurance.

The following comfort measures may make an asthma attack more tolerable or help it subside. Strengthening the child's health between attacks can decrease their frequency and severity, and is the best prevention for asthma attacks. But when attacks do occur, and they may continue even after herbal treatment has begun, you should not hesitate to use medical help. A simple medical intervention is preferable to waiting until your child is in danger.

- *Encourage relaxation:* As we relax, our breathing passages open to receive more air. Teach your child to get into a comfortable position, loosen any clothing around the collar and waist, and practice a guided visualization to relax the muscles of the neck, face, chest, and belly. Any imagery that your child finds relaxing is appropriate. Everyone around the child should remain as calm as possible, breathing deeply themselves. Panic is contagious and will only aggravate the child and worsen the situation. Even a trip to the hospital need not be frantic. Many useful books on visualization and meditation for children are available (see "Further Reading"); some titles include *Meditating with Children,* by Deborah Rozman; *Spinning Inward: Using Guided Imagery with Children,* by Maureen Murdock; and *Motherwit,* by Diane Marieschild. Help your child become familiar with visualization and meditation techniques before an attack. See the accompanying box for a simple visualization that you can use any time your child needs help relaxing.
- *Change the environment:* If the room is hot and stuffy, let in some fresh air or take the child outdoors (dressed to avoid chill). If the air is very dry, turn your bathroom into a sauna by shutting the door and turning on the hot-water faucets until the room is quite steamy. If the child begins to feel some relief, stay with him in this room as long as necessary until he is breathing normally. A few drops of thyme or eucalyptus oil in a pot of hot water will enhance the benefits of the moist air. A bath with 1/2 teaspoon of thyme oil added may be particularly soothing for babies and very young children.
- *Provide fluids:* Rapid breathing can cause dehydration. Drinking plenty of fluids prevents dehydration and helps loosen excess mucus, easing the breathing difficulty. Do not give any cold drinks to the child. Serve lots of room-temperature or slightly warm water, and let the child sip on herbal teas.
- *Give massage:* During an asthma attack, massage can encourage your child to relax his chest and can also take the focus off the breathing difficulty. Specific massage techniques also stimulate

channels in the body that correlate to the lungs, enabling the attack to subside more easily. Use the following steps as a series, or just use the parts you find most useful. Practice giving your child a massage between attacks to become confident with the techniques.

1. *Feet:* Have the child get into a semi-reclining position, supported from behind by either a lot of pillows or another adult. Be certain that the air in the room is fresh and that the child is covered and comfortably warm. Your own hands should be warm, too. Begin by uncovering one foot. Hold the foot in one hand; starting at the heel, press the thumb of your other hand inward with a moderate amount of pressure. Hold for three to five seconds; then release. Using the same motion, work your way slowly and steadily toward this big toe. Return to the heel and repeat until you reach the top of the second toe, and so on until you have massaged the whole foot. Next rub the soft areas behind and beneath the ankles, and massage each toe. Cover the foot and put it down gently. Repeat the entire sequence on the other foot.

2. *Back:* The child should sit facing outward in the lap of the person doing the massage or sit backward with legs straddling the chair so he can lean his head and shoulders onto its backrest. A young child may sit backward straddling the lap of a seated parent, resting against his or her chest for support while the other parent massages the back. It is preferable to do this with the child's shirt off if the air is warm enough. A light massage oil containing ginger, calendula, or thyme oil or relaxing herbs such as lavender, chamomile, or St. John's wort may be used. The oil should be warmed in your hands.

   Begin by gently placing your hands on the child's shoulders at the base of the neck. Using your palms, gently rub outward over the shoulders about ten times. Next, extend your thumbs and place them just below the level of the shoulder blades in toward the spine, about a half inch from it on either side. Place the rest of your fingers and palms gently but firmly on the back to support your thumbs. Apply even pressure inward and slightly upward for about ten seconds every half inch along the sides of the spine. Now release pressure slightly and slide your thumbs outward toward the shoulder blades, maintaining moderate pressure as you do so. Return to the starting position and repeat this technique until you reach the shoulders. Apply gentle pressure downward at the halfway point between the neck and outer edge of the shoulders.

The child may find this massage slightly uncomfortable at first, so be responsive to his reactions, and yet persistent because it will facilitate deep relaxation and thus reduce breathing difficulty. For more on massage techniques for children when they are ill, refer to *Turtle Tail and Other Tender Mercies: Traditional Chinese Pediatrics*, by Bob Flaws, and *Natural Medicine for Children*, by Julian Scott (see "Further Reading").

3. *Chest and arm massage:* This can be done with the child either upright or lying down. For chest massage, run your hands (with your fingers outstretched) horizontally from the center of the rib cage to the outer area of the rib cage. Apply firm but light pressure, taking care not to tickle the child. If using the fingertips causes tickling, use the palms of your hands instead. For arm massage, apply firm inward pressure as you use your fingers and hands to gently squeeze along the length of the arm from just below the underarm to the wrist. Next, use your thumbs and fingertips to massage the hand and fingers.

HERBAL RECOMMENDATIONS

Many herbalists recommend the following remedies for use during asthma attacks. They are strong acting, so the child should be watched for the adverse side effects mentioned below. If these are seen, just discontinue usage, and there will be no long-term problems. Do not use for children too young to alert you to unpleasant reactions. If your child continues to have severe attacks despite these remedies, seek the support of an experienced practitioner as well as consulting a physician.

- *Lobelia inflata:* Early American herbalists commonly used lobelia to dispel an asthma attack. Known also as "puke-weed," lobelia has emetic properties that encourage expectoration of mucus and antispasmodic properties that encourage relaxation of the lungs and ease difficult breathing.

  Homeopathic Lobelia inflata 30x: Taken as needed through the onset of an attack, this remedy may be used with no side effects.

Lobelia tincture: Give 1/4–2 teaspoons depending on the age of the child. If no side effects are seen, repeat as needed no more than every thirty minutes for a few hours. Side effects include tight, scratching, or burning throat; stupor; and nausea.

Lobelia and catnip infusion: Steep one small handful of each herb in a quart of boiling water for thirty minutes. Serve hot, 1/4 to 1/2 cup at a time, as needed, watching for side effects for fifteen minutes before repeating the dosage.

- *Ephedra and catnip tea:* Ephedra, also known as "Mormon tea," and related to the stronger species Chinese ephedra (Ma Huang), is an old lung remedy shared with us by Native Americans. It is a powerful bronchial dilator and stimulant so those already on medications as well as those with heart problems, high blood pressure, or thyroid or kidney problems should completely avoid its use. Joy Gardner (1989) suggests monitoring the child's heartbeat for thirty minutes after using ephedra. To do this, seat the child in your lap with your hand over his heart or listen with your ear over his chest and count the beats for one minute (use a watch with a second hand to keep track of the time as you count). Repeat this periodically during the thirty minutes. For children between one and seven years, the average heartbeat is 80 to 120 beats per minute. In children over seven years, it is 80 to 90 beats. If using the ephedra remedy causes the heart rate to exceed the normal range, discontinue and give catnip or lemon balm tea or 15 drops of valerian tincture to restore calm.

  To prepare, simmer 1 ounce dry ephedra in 1 quart water in a covered pot for twenty minutes. Turn off the heat and add 1/4 ounce catnip or lemon balm leaves. Steep ten more minutes. Sweeten if necessary. Give 1 teaspoon to 2 tablespoons at a time depending on age. Wait a half hour between doses. You may give up to 1 cup a day to children over seven, less to very young children, but follow the above precautions.

CARE BETWEEN ASTHMA ATTACKS

The main goal of this section is to encourage you to strengthen your child's health and alter your environment between attacks in order to eliminate their underlying cause and prevent recurrence as much as possible. In addition to the following suggestions, counseling may be helpful to address emotional issues if you suspect that attacks may be related to them.

DIET

Do your best to remove any suspected allergens from your diet. If you are uncertain about what your child is allergic to, a health practitioner in your area can teach you how to identify them. There are also many books on allergies.

Diets stressing natural foods are important in the reduction of health problems and will help your child establish lifelong habits that may reduce the incidence of other illnesses. You needn't make extreme changes in your diet, but you can substitute natural ingredients for synthetic ones as a start, and begin to incorporate new dishes into your menus.

Children with asthma benefit from a diet free of cold-natured foods. These include any foods eaten straight from the refrigerator, foods that come from tropical climates (unless you live in one), and fruits that are out of season. Asthmatic children also benefit from a small amount of meat added to the diet on a regular basis.

MASSAGE

The massage described earlier for acute attacks may be used every other day between attacks to both strengthen your child and prevent recurrence. Eventually once a week will be sufficient. Massage is a healing family ritual that children will cherish, whether asthmatic or not. Acupuncture may be a useful therapy for treating asthma, but be cautious in your choice of practitioners for young children. Acupressure can be used similarly to acupuncture and requires a less extensively trained practitioner.

HERBS

The following brews may be used as is, or in your own personal combinations, to encourage lung and digestive strength as well as general immunity. The child should drink at least one recommended dosage of the chosen formula each day.

- *Respiratory tonic tea:* This recipe, developed by Rosemary Gladstar Slick (*Herbs for Children*), is my favorite because it is both effective and delicious, a big help in formulas for kids. She regards it as "especially helpful for children who have recurring respiratory problems such as colds, flus, hayfever, asthma, ear infections, and general congestion." It is intended to be "used over a period of time to aid in creating a healthy respiratory system." Mix the following dried herbs: 1 ounce each of red clover flowers and comfrey leaves, 1/2 ounce each of calendula flowers, mullein leaves, coltsfoot, lemon grass, and rosehips; and 1/4 ounce fennel seeds. Make an infusion of 1/2 ounce of the mix to 1 quart water. Give between 1/2 cup and 2 cups daily depending on the child's age.

A SAMPLE VISUALIZATION

The following visualization is a small example of what is possible to share with a child who for whatever reason is restless, uncomfortable, or ill. Before you begin the visualization (also called "guided imagery"), set the mood by dimming the lights or closing the curtains, putting on quiet instrumental music if available, and helping the child get comfortable. Speak in soft, dreamy tones and allow for pauses between sentences as you weave a richly textured "story" in which your child can drift off. Keep weaving the story or images until you see that your little one is restful. Of course, always be careful to avoid words or images that may be frightening—anything having to do with separation from you, darkness, or death, as it would obviously be counterproductive.

"Get comfortable in bed. Fluff your pillow up nice and soft. Pull your covers around you. There, are you feeling more comfortable now? Good. Close your eyes, and I will be here as you relax.

Let's pretend we are in a meadow. A beautiful emerald green meadow filled with wild flowers of many colors. There are yellow, pink, blue, and violet flowers as far as your eyes can see. And there is a soft, sweet fragrance in the air. Let's go to the center of the meadow and sit down. Good. Oh, this grass is so soft. I could just stretch right out into it as if it were a bed made of feathers. Go ahead, let yourself lay back in the soft grass, and feel yourself surrounded by the scent and colors of the flowers. Mmmm. Feel the warm sun on your face and the slight breeze in the air. Birds are softly chirping, and you can hear the faint rustle of the leaves from the trees at the edge of the meadow. What a perfect day.

"Just above you in the clear blue sky you begin to notice a small cloud beginning to form. It is growing just a little larger, and you can see that it is more than a cloud—it is a castle. A castle in the sky. And there is a long spiral staircase slowly unfolding. Down, down the staircase you see floating the loveliest little butterfly you could ever imagine. She glides down the staircase until she is fluttering just next to you. You look at her, and as you are looking, she becomes a lovely and gentle woman with golden light shimmering all about her. She takes your hand in one of hers, and with the other she strokes your brow. She speaks your name in quiet whispers, telling you that you are filled with the light and health of all the world. She tells you that the peacefulness of the meadow is within you, that the beauty of the flowers is within you, and that the blessing of love is all around you. She sits beside you as you rest peacefully, knowing that you will wake refreshed and loved."

If by now your child has become restful or has fallen asleep, slowly lower the tone of your voice so that stopping doesn't abruptly awaken him or her. If he or she is on the verge of sleep, continue to embellish the imagery until the child is resting fully.

- *Elecampane infusion:* To 1/4 ounce elecampane add 1/4 ounce of any of the following: comfrey leaves, chickweed, burdock root, fenugreek seeds, anise seeds, or other herbs beneficial to the lungs. Steep in 1 quart boiling water for one hour. Strain, sweeten, and refrigerate the extra. Dosage is 1/4 to 1 cup daily depending on the child's age. A teaspoon of ephedra may be added to the steeping herbs if your child is having frequent attacks.
- *Violet tea:* On a beautiful spring day you can easily gather the herbs for this tea. The activity of harvesting wild violets is so pleasant that I encourage you to venture outdoors with basket in hand every available afternoon.

  Use this gentle tonic for the lungs in addition to the teas already mentioned, or add violets to elecampane infusion. To prepare as a tea, steep one handful of violet leaves and blossoms (heavy on the leaves)—discard roots as they are too strong for general use—in 1 cup boiling water for a half hour. Strain and drink.

❖ BED-WETTING ❖

Bed-wetting (*enuresis* in medical terminology) rarely requires medical attention because usually no physiological problem exists. But for both the child and parents it is a big inconvenience. It is uncomfortable for the child to be wet and cold and to have his or her sleep interrupted; it is also embarrassing, particularly when the child wants to spend the night with a friend. And, of course, there is the extra laundry.

Common among boys, bed-wetting is almost always outgrown by the early teenage years. Frequently, boys who are bed-wetters have dads who were bed-wetters around the same age. While you may choose to consult with a physician, be cautious about taking drastic measures like surgery.

No matter what the reason for bed-wetting, avoid chastising the child no matter how frustrated you feel. It is hard enough for your child without being scolded, too. Instead, there are many positive things you can do to strengthen your child and minimize and perhaps eliminate bed-wetting.

GENERAL RECOMMENDATIONS

- *Strengthen the bladder:* The muscle that we release to allow our urine to flow is called the "urethral sphincter." It can be released both voluntarily and involuntarily, and through a simple exercise it can be strengthened. This exercise, known as "the Kegel" (named after the doctor who demonstrated the benefits of it for pregnant women), is helpful for all people. It reduces urinary incontinence, a common but preventable problem in our society. Teach your children this exercise while young, and they are more likely to avoid incontinence problems later in life.

To teach your child to recognize the sphincter, have him or her stop the flow of urine midstream, and then release it again. Practicing during the day both while urinating and when not will greatly increase bladder control. Have your child do the exercise ten times a day at first. For bed-wetting, work up to fifty times a day after a few weeks of practice. Each contraction of the muscle can be held to a count of five seconds. Try having the child pretend that the muscle is an elevator being lifted up into the body one floor at a time up to the fifth floor. The muscle is then released back to the first floor. You can encourage your child to use this exercise during the night to stop the flow of urine when he feels the urge to pee and to hold it until he gets to the bathroom.

- *Strengthen the kidneys:* Bed-wetting may be due to kidney weakness, a condition often accompanied by a general chilliness, cold hands and feet, a pale complexion, and sometimes fatigue and loss of appetite. To strengthen the kidneys, you will need to bring warmth to your child's body, particularly in the area of the child's kidneys and bladder. Here are some ways to do this.

  Clothing: Keep your child's lower back and abdomen warm by having him wear a cotton thermal undershirt and teaching him to keep it tucked in. A wool vest or sweater worn over the clothing also affords extra warmth.

  Moxibustion: This is the application of heat to specific areas of the body by holding a lit moxa stick, a "cigar" made of Chinese mugwort, just above the skin. When applied properly, the heat is penetrating without burning. This is a simple, effective method for tonifying the kidneys and bladder. You can purchase moxa sticks through the mail from suppliers of herbal products (see "Resources"). Also available are "little smoke moxa sticks" that generate less smoke.

  To use the moxa stick, unwrap and remove the outer paper, leaving the inner wrapper in place. Working in a room that is well ventilated but not too drafty, light the tip of the moxa stick and let it burn until it is glowing red hot. You may need to blow on it to get it glowing. Have the child lying comfortable in bed, and keep an ashtray or a dish nearby to hold ashes or the roll should you need to set it down.

  Heat should be directed as follows: On the abdomen you will warm an area that forms the shape of an equilateral triangle with the apex just above the pubic bone and the base just below the navel. The area should be about as wide as the child's own outstretched hand. On the child's back you will warm a corresponding triangular area that extends from just above the sacrum and over the small of the back.

Uncover the area to be heated. Holding the moxa stick in your hand as you would a pencil, position the glowing end about 1 to 2 inches above the treatment spot and begin moving it circularly in small areas about 2 inches in diameter. Periodically knock any accumulated ashes into the dish. When the child tells you the spot is getting warm, move to the next small area. By working in small adjacent areas you will eventually cover the whole region. Treat until the whole region is warm but not uncomfortably hot. The skin may become pink but should not be red or burnt. *NEVER give a moxibustion treatment to anyone who cannot tell you very clearly that his skin is becoming too hot!* This includes young children not yet talking, anyone asleep or unconscious, or anyone on pain medication.

To extinguish the moxa stick, you can insert it into a specially designed moxa extinguisher (these are inexpensive and can be purchased through suppliers listed in "Resources"), you can smother it in a dish of sand, or you can run the tip through water for a few seconds. Don't leave it in a dish unextinguished as it tends to smoulder.

Moxibustion can be continued for many months, particularly during cold weather. Do not use the technique if the child has any infections at the time.

- *Limit fluids:* Encourage your child to drink plenty of fluids early in the day. Discourage drinking after 5 P.M.
- *Counseling and understanding:* Sometimes bed-wetting has its basis in emotional or psychological upsets. For example, a four- or five-year-old may begin to wet the bed after the birth of a sibling as a way of "being the baby" and getting that extra attention he or she is craving. Something disturbing may be going on at school or at home that is causing your child to suppress fear or anger. When bed-wetting is a problem with boys, the father-son relationship may need nurturing and healing. If you suspect underlying issues, a counselor can be of service when you are unable to get to the root of the problem.

Herbal Recommendations

- Corn silk tea is the most reputable herb for helping with bed-wetting. Make an infusion using 2 ounces of corn silk (preferably fresh and from organic corn) to 1 quart water. Steep for one hour and strain. Give the tea early in the day. The dose is 1/2 cup twice daily.
- Other herbs considered beneficial for bladder problems are horsetail, rosemary, and parsley. One-quarter ounce of any of these herbs, alone or in combination, may be added to the corn silk brew.
- Celery (yes, the vegetable) is also a urinary-tract tonic. Encourage your child to eat fresh celery daily. It is also a nervous-system tonic.
- Many Chinese herbal formulas are intended to strengthen the kidneys. The specific formula and dosage is based on the individual child's constitutional type and accompanying symptoms. If you wish to use this approach, which has been used in China for over two thousand years, I refer you to *Turtle Tail and Other Tender Mercies: Traditional Chinese Pediatrics*, by Bob Flaws (see "Further Reading").

❖ Bites and Stings ❖

For children who enjoy playing outdoors, insect bites and even an occasional bee sting are an inevitable fact of life. Provided that your child is not allergic to any particular insect venom, the following remedies should provide sufficient relief of the symptoms.

WHEN TO SEEK MEDICAL CARE

Any child with a known allergy should receive appropriate medical attention. Even children with no previous history of allergy can develop a dangerous allergic reaction. Any breathing difficulty, signs of shock, significant swelling, or other unusual reactions require immediate attention. Poisonous snake and spider bites need to be evaluated quickly on an individual basis as do bites from wild animals and even domestic pets: seek emergency medical care.

Ant Bites

The venom of red ants has varying degrees of reaction depending on a person's sensitivity. Reactions range from an itchy fluid-filled vesicle the size of a pinhead to localized swelling, fever, and general discomfort. Young children generally seem to get the worst bites because they may be standing on an anthill for some time before noticing that they are covered with ants and are being bitten. It is difficult for children to get all the ants off by themselves, and the ants will continue to bite in a frenzy. If you know red ants live in your vicinity, teach children to recognize anthills and to stay away from them.

Treatment: Get all the ants off! Wash the bites with apple cider vinegar. Then apply a thin slip of green clay or healing salve. Alternatively, a plantain poultice can be used. Echinacea tincture may be given internally for inflammation and mild reactions. For extensive bites, give the child a cool bath with apple cider vinegar or baking soda (1/2 cup per bath).

BEE STINGS

To avoid bee stings, teach your child not to panic around bees, to just move slowly and calmly away.

If your child does get stung, first remove the stinger if it is still in the skin. Hold and comfort your child and give Bach Rescue Remedy or Calm Child Formula (see "Car Sickness"). Stings are surprising and frightening, and initially can be quite painful. As soon as possible, chew up a fresh plantain leaf and apply it as a poultice onto the bite to draw out the poison and discomfort. Repeat this as often as necessary. Plantain is available in most parts of the United States from spring through autumn. Unsurpassed in treating bites and stings, it has many other uses and is easy to identify. If you don't have plantain, tobacco or mud are also effective in treating bee stings. Other remedies include apple cider vinegar, calendula oil, and green clay.

Give repeated oral doses of echinacea tincture, plantain tincture, and vitamin C. They are anti-inflammatory, meaning they reduce swelling, and prevent systemic poisoning.

WHEN TO SEEK MEDICAL CARE

If you know your child is allergic to bee stings, or if your child shows signs of an allergic reaction to a bee sting, seek immediate medical help. Don't waste any time! Localized swelling, itching, and pain are all normal reactions to a sting. Difficulty breathing, generalized swelling, extreme anxiety, signs of shock, or other unusual responses may be signs of an allergic reaction.

Epinephrine, an antihistamine used to counteract allergic reactions to bee stings, is available in easy-to-use kits at pharmacies (you may need a prescription). If you suspect your child is allergic to bee stings, you may want to keep it in your first-aid kit.

Dog Bites

While most household dogs and wild animals will not harm children, a bite can confer serious infection. The primary infection that poses a risk is rabies. Teach children basic safety by telling them not to approach any dog from behind to pet it, stay away from unfamiliar animals, not to pet a dog without the owner's permission, and should a strange or aggressive dog approach him or her, not to run away but to stay stationary and then back away slowly. Healthy wild animals tend to shy away from people while rabid animals may actually approach people. Teach children not to pick up or pet any wild animals such as squirrels, chipmunks, or any rodents, as well as larger animals such as foxes. While most pets are protected by the rabies vaccine, which prevents them from transmitting the disease, many wild animals are carriers and not all pets kept are up-to-date with their shots.

If you have any suspicion that your child was bitten by a rabid animal, seek medical advice quickly. An unprovoked attack, an animal that is acting strange, or an unknown animal should be considered suspect. The standard medical treatment is advisable and must begin before signs of the illness develop. Your county animal-control officer can help you determine whether the animal was in fact rabid, and give you information on the risks of the disease occurring in your area.

If the animal bite results in a puncture wound, your child may be at risk for tetanus. If your child is unvaccinated, you will have to evaluate the necessity for giving the tetanus toxoid based upon the type of wound, your child's health, and your overall assessment of the situation. Consultation with a medical or naturopathic practitioner is highly advisable. If tetanus seems to be a significant concern, the risk of the disease outweighs the risk of a reaction to the vaccine. Reactions to the vaccine as well as the tetanus toxoid are rare and usually occur only after many doses.

Immediate treatment for any animal bite is to thoroughly wash the area under running water with a mild soap. Let water run over the area, flushing it completely, for about ten minutes. Some bleeding is good because it helps clean the wound from the inside out. Allow the wound to bleed a little bit while running the area under water. Of course, excessive bleeding needs to be controlled, which can be done by applying firm pressure to the wound for a few minutes. Rinse with a strong infusion of rosemary and calendula (1 ounce each to 2 quarts water) or diluted tinctures of these herbs. Alternatives are rue, wormwood, thyme, and apple cider vinegar. Hydrogen peroxide is useful for cleaning out wounds and serves the additional function of aerating the site. This is particularly beneficial if tetanus is a concern because its spores can thrive only in an anaerobic (nonoxygenated) environment. Leave the wound open or covered only with a light gauze to keep out dirt. This will also allow air to reach the area.

Internally give Bach Rescue Remedy or other relaxing herbs for stress and fright. Immediately give echinacea tincture, 1 drop per 2 pounds of body weight, and repeat every few hours. Calendula tincture can be given in addition, about 5 to 15 drops every few hours.

If home care has been deemed adequate, repeat the washing procedure for a few minutes four times each day. Allow the wound to stay moist, and encourage healing from the inside out. In other words, don't let a scab form over the top of the wound until the puncture or laceration has healed below the surface. Continue to give the internal remedies every few hours for three days; then decrease to a couple of times a day until the wound has scabbed over.

If any signs of infection develop, consult the section on abscesses, and follow the recommendations *and* precautions detailed there.

MOSQUITO AND OTHER ITCHY BUG BITES

Apply healing salve, aloe vera gel, calendula oil, green clay, plantain poultices, chickweed poultices, or witch hazel (the drugstore preparation is fine for this use). Repeat as needed. Cool baths are relieving. Encourage kids not to scratch or pick at bites, keeping their fingernails short if necessary. For infected mosquito bites refer to "Impetigo."

SNAKE AND SPIDER BITES

You and your children should know how to identify the snakes in your vicinity. Even in the middle of Atlanta, Georgia, we have both poisonous snakes and poisonous spiders. Teach children respect for all wild creatures, and they are not likely to get hurt. They can be taught where snakes live and not to put their hands and feet in burrows; under rocks, logs, or boards; or in holes. They should also know that when faced with one of these creatures, they should not panic; they should just slowly and calmly move away. Refer to field guides and your local nature centers for information. Naturalists generally enjoy sharing what they know.

Treatment of poisonous bites depends upon the animal, the age of the person bitten, and the location of the bite on the body. The following are emergency measures you should take until medical help is available. Nonpoisonous bites may also be quite painful.

Some snakes, such as the cottonmouth water moccasin, are more poisonous than others. The venom of some spiders (like the brown recluse) can cause significant damage to the area surrounding the bite, while the venom of others (like the black widow) can cause systemic collapse. Young children have small bodies and quick metabolism, so venom may affect them more quickly than older kids or adults. The closer the bite is to the heart, the more dangerous the situation. In all cases your careful judgment is required.

WHEN TO SEEK MEDICAL CARE

If your child is bitten by a poisonous snake or spider, seek emergency assistance.

1. *Encourage the child to be as still and calm as possible.* This will delay the spread of the venom through the body and give you a chance to assess the situation. Give Bach Rescue Remedy, 4 drops repeated as often as necessary, or homeopathic arnica 30x every fifteen minutes to prevent shock and treat the fear. Skullcap, valerian, or St. John's wort can be used to promote calm and prevent hysteria.

2. *Discourage the spread of the venom.* Apply an ice pack to the bite and the surrounding area. This is the preferable and safest way to slow the circulation and localize the poison.

The "cut-and-suck" method and the "tourniquet" method for treating bites are well known and can be effective. Each, however, poses significant risks. The cut-and-suck method exposes the bite victim to risk of infection from the cut and can cause the person sucking the venom to be poisoned. This method is actually out of favor but may be helpful as a last result. The tourniquet method cuts off circulation to and from the area, which could lead to the loss of the appendage on which the tourniquet was tied. Either method may be preferable to none in an emergency situation occurring in a remote area far from medical assistance. If you must use a tourniquet, be certain to loosen it at least every ten minutes and then completely as soon as better options become available.

3. *Use appropriate remedies.* If you need to use antivenom serum, you must go to a hospital or clinic that has it available. If you live in or travel to a high-risk area, it may be worth your while to find out which facilities keep it in stock.

All bites in young children merit medical attention. For bites that are mild enough to treat at home, you can use the following herbal allies:

INTERNAL REMEDIES

- For pain, use tinctures or infusions of skullcap, valerian, St. John's wort, lobelia, or Bach Rescue Remedy as needed to help the child rest without masking the body's symptoms. Pain is normal, but extreme pain is the body's way of asking for help.

- For eliminating the poison, give frequent doses (as often as every one to two hours) of echinacea and plantain infusion or tinctures. The number of drops of echinacea tincture should be equal to the child's body weight in pounds. Give 20 drops of plantain tincture or 1/4 cup of infusion (use fresh leaves) each time.
- Give plenty of water.
- Chickweed, burdock root, and violet leaf infusions reduce inflammation. Let the child sip on an infusion made of equal parts of these herbs, up to a quart daily.

EXTERNAL REMEDIES

- Alternate between poultices of plantain and thin layers of green clay, keeping one or the other constantly applied to the wound. Change the dressings as soon as they become warm. A few times a day apply compresses of chickweed, burdock root, or violet leaves.

❖ BOILS ❖

A boil is an acute local inflammation of the skin, a gland, or a hair follicle. Most often they are due to invasion of staph bacteria. Most boils can be treated with hot compresses. Medical treatment for boils is to prescribe antibiotics; if the boil does not drain on its own, then it is lanced, meaning an incision is made to allow it to drain. This is done under local anesthetic at a physician's office, unless the infection is severe and deep.

WHEN TO SEEK MEDICAL CARE

Signs of infection that indicate the need for more rigorous treatment include red streaks emanating from the boil, persistent fever, generalized boils, or general illness. If you see these signs, seek further help promptly.

Home treatment consists of a combination of internal and external herbal remedies and moist heat, similar to the approach for abscesses. Boils can become quite large and angry looking, but as long as your child is in good health with no signs of general infection, you can continue with home remedies.

When the boil opens, it is important to keep the area very clean and to prevent the infected pus from contacting other areas of the body or anyone else. *Staphylococcus* is highly contagious. Thoroughly wash the area under running water twice a day, and launder any bedding, wash cloths, or towels if they have become contaminated. If you have touched the open wound or otherwise had contact with it, thoroughly wash your hands.

Some boils are resistant to draining on their own even after they become large and appear "ripe." In this case, the herbs, applied regularly, will soften the boil enough to allow it to be merely stuck with a large-gauge needle by your physician without local anesthetic. The procedure should be only momentarily uncomfortable for your child. You and your physician can together determine the severity of the infection and whether your child requires antibiotics. If not, you can continue the internal recommendations for abscesses to heal the infection and prevent reinfection.

GENERAL RECOMMENDATIONS

- Keep the area surrounding the boil very clean.
- The child should avoid any rough activities that can result in impact to the boil as this can be painful and add insult to injury. In addition, he or she should be encouraged to get extra rest.
- Apply heat to the boil, preferably via herbal compresses, many times a day.

DIETARY RECOMMENDATIONS

- Follow recommendations for abscesses.
- The child should drink *plenty* of fluids.

HERBAL RECOMMENDATIONS

The internal herbal treatment for boils is exactly the same as for abscesses and should be followed diligently along with these external treatments:

- Apply hot herbal compresses up to every two hours, the frequency depending upon the severity of the boil. Compresses should be as hot as tolerable and applied for twenty minutes each time. Excellent herbal choices for boils include infusions of burdock root, chickweed, violet leaves, and plantain leaves, alone or in combination.
- In between compresses, apply poultices to draw out or resolve the infection. Powdered herbs can be mixed with water to form a paste; leaves or roots can be finely grated or chopped and applied as is or mixed with herbal powder and then applied. Choose from the following herbs and vegetables: plantain leaves, burdock root, grated raw potato, green clay, green cabbage leaves, slippery elm powder, beet root, and fenugreek seeds.

- After the boil opens and drains, wash the area and sprinkle a mixture of equal parts of myrrh, echinacea, and chaparral powders into the wound. This will check the infection and absorb any drainage. Apply hot compresses twice a day until all drainage ceases and the swelling completely subsides. This process may require a couple of days to complete. (If chaparral is unavailable, either omit it or substitute goldenseal powder.)
- The Chinese herb astragalus (which can be grown in the United States) is specifically used for nourishing the immune system. After the boil has healed, continue to give your child between 10 and 25 drops of astragalus root tincture twice a day for two to three weeks. This will boost your child's health and prevent further infection.

❖ BROKEN BONES ❖

With all the sports activities children are involved in, and all the physical feats they need to accomplish (like defying gravity!), it's no wonder kids sometimes break bones. Of course, strong bones and a healthy dose of carefulness will go a long way in preventing most fractures, but an occasional accident is inevitable.

Frequently, broken bones do not need emergency medical treatment. The exceptions are broken ribs, fractures in which the bone has punctured through the skin, and elbow and thigh fractures, which can lead to internal hemorrhaging with nerve damage and loss of blood supply to the extremities. Fractures in children are usually less dramatic than this, so you can take a little time to calm your child and yourself and assess the situation.

When you suspect that the child has broken a bone, help him or her into a comfortable position with the injured part supported by a pillow. The child is likely to instinctively immobilize the injured part, much as a splint would do. Because the pain of a fracture can be severe, it may cause the child to faint, so be sure that he or she is situated securely. Pain this severe indicates a serious injury, and the damage should be medically evaluated without delay.

After the initial fright has subsided, if your child remains in constant pain, is totally unable to get comfortable, seems unable to move the affected or surrounding areas, consult with a medical care provider. Some fractures must be set to ensure that the bones continue to grow properly as they heal. The use of x-rays will be necessary for this. Two x-rays should be sufficient for most simple breaks: one before and one after setting the bone. If appropriate, try to obtain some form of removable cast because it allows for the regular application of external remedies.

Sometimes minor fractures can be successfully treated at home without the use of x-rays and casts.

GENERAL AND DIETARY RECOMMENDATIONS

- Plenty of rest is essential for the healing of traumatic injuries. Encourage your child to be patient with the healing process. Some things just take time.
- *Gentle* massage of the area surrounding the fracture along with the external treatments that follow facilitate blood flow to the area and ensure that the muscles retain their strength. Massage is a form of passive exercise that greatly aids healing. Consult with your health care provider as to when it would be appropriate to begin.
- When the child seems ready, begin gentle exercises that rebuild the strength of the muscles that have been at rest for many weeks.
- If your child is on crutches, help him resist the temptation to be overly active. It is important to honor our bodies' limitations and respect the time needed for healing.
- Healing a fracture requires a lot of high-quality vitamins, minerals, and protein to rebuild bone and surrounding tissue. A diet rich in vegetables, especially dark leafy greens (kale, collards, broccoli, mustard greens), orange vegetables (carrots, squash, and sweet potatoes), seafoods (fish and seaweeds), fresh fruits, and seeds and nuts will help build the bones.

HERBAL RECOMMENDATIONS

Treating broken bones with herbs involves three approaches: providing pain relief, boosting the child's mineral intake, helping to heal damaged tissue. How much to emphasize each approach depends on the severity of the injury. Please bear in mind that you are not trying to totally eliminate pain because it is an important signal that lets you know how healing is progressing. Nor do you want to eliminate pain to the point that the child is able to do things that he or she isn't yet ready to do. The pain helps keep activity to a minimum. You are just trying to take the edge off the discomfort so that the child is able to rest comfortably and adequately.

- Nervine herbs provide calming pain relief at the outset of the break and thereafter. You can use chamomile, catnip, and lemon balm teas; in addition, give 5 to 20 drops of skullcap, St. John's wort, or valerian tinctures. The tinctures can be repeated every thirty minutes, and the tea can be given freely.

- Homeopathic arnica 30x should be given every fifteen to thirty minutes for the first couple of hours to minimize bruising, fright, and anxiety.
- If there have been no skin abrasions, arnica oil can be rubbed gently onto the area of the break.
- To supplement calcium and other minerals to heal the fracture, as well as to provide astringency and allantoin, which creates the fiber that knits the bones back together, give your child the following infusion: *Bone-Fusion:* Mix together 1 ounce each of nettles, oatstraw, and comfrey leaves; 1/2 ounce each of horsetail, skullcap, and marshmallow root; and 1/4 ounce each of fennel seeds and peppermint leaves. Infuse 1 ounce of the mixture in 1 quart of boiling water for thirty minutes. Dosage is 2 cups daily. It can be sweetened if desired.
- Chamomile, red raspberry leaves, and slippery elm bark are also high in calcium and can be used as teas for variety. It is interesting to note that these and many herbs that provide pain relief are calcium rich.
- "BF & C" (Bone, Flesh, and Cartilage) is a packaged formula developed by the late herbalist Dr. John Christopher that combines the properties of astringency, high nutrient content, and nerve calming. Available in many natural-food stores in capsule form, it is indicated for fractures. Use according to the directions on the package. It is also available as a cream for external application.
- Externally use frequent soaks or compresses of comfrey leaf and root infusion, up to four times a day. In addition, apply oils of arnica (as long as no skin is broken), calendula, or St. John's wort a few times a day.
- For optimal tonification, maintain dietary and external herbal treatments for a couple of weeks after the fracture has completely healed.

❖ BRUISES ❖

Bumps and bruises are a fact of life in a healthy, active childhood, so I always keep 1 ounce bottles of arnica oil and calendula oil on hand. Arnica is amazing. Rubbed onto a bruise or bump, it immediately reduces pain and swelling (however, it should never be applied to broken skin). Topical applications of calendula or St. John's wort oil may be used. Compresses of comfrey leaf are also helpful. Homeopathic *Arnica montana* 30x can be given internally for all injuries, especially bruises.

Children who bruise easily may have nutritional deficiencies and may benefit from vitamin C with bioflavinoids (also called vitamin P, these substances found in fruits and vegetables occur with vitamin C and greatly enhance its absorption; they also maintain the walls of small blood vessels). Citrus fruits eaten with the white part of the skin still attached, buckwheat, and fresh leafy green vegetables are important sources of these nutrients.

WHEN TO SEEK MEDICAL CARE

For severe, chronic and easy (as compared to other children for example) bruising problems, seek an experienced caregiver's help, to determine the existence of underlying disease.

❖ BURNS ❖

Burns are painful and can cause lasting damage. The best treatment for them is prevention. Keep hot objects well out of a child's reach; even a baby or toddler can reach the edge of a tabletop and pull over hot soup or a hot beverage. I know one woman who left a cup of coffee on the floor and her four-year-old stepped in it, incurring a painful burn. Minor burns are inevitable as children learn important skills such as food preparation and lighting matches, but basic precautions should prevent most serious injuries.

See below for immediate emergency treatment at home. In the case of serious burns, however, home treatment is not a substitute for medical care.

Burns that are red but do not form blisters are considered "first-degree burns." These are minor burns but can still be quite painful. Run the affected part under cool water. If you have some, a piece of tofu placed on the burn draws out the heat. For healing and pain relief, apply calendula oil or ointment as needed. Calendula is an incredible herb for healing burns, attending to both the pain and the burn with a loving hand. It should always be kept in the home medicine chest. Aloe vera gel is also effective for soothing burns, so you may want to keep an aloe plant in your home. To use it, cut a piece of the plant and rub the cut edge on the affected area.

WHEN TO SEEK MEDICAL CARE

Emergency medical care is required for all burns that cover an area on the body larger than twice the size of the child's hand, if there are any signs of shock, or if the burn site becomes infected.

"Second-degree burns" also become very red, but the area will blister and appear bubbly. The water that collects under the skin nourishes the damaged area. Do not pop the blisters. If the blisters open or if the area of the burn is dirty, gently wash the burn with clean, cool water and a mild soap. Immediately move clothing away from the burn and apply cool water until the area feels cool. Next, apply calendula oil or ointment, raw honey, or aloe vera gel to a clean sterile gauze or linen and drape over the burn. Localized second-degree burns can usually be treated well at home, but they must be kept clean and watched for signs of infection. If the burn covers a large area of the body, medical treatment should be sought without hesitation.

Change the gauze twice a day, gently rinsing the area if it has become dirty. Any sign of infection (pus, swelling, general illness, fever, or swollen lymph nodes) means you need to treat for infection as well as the burn (see "Abscesses"). Again, if the healing extends beyond your confidence and experience level, seek medical care promptly.

WHEN TO SEEK MEDICAL CARE

In a "third-degree burn," the surface layers of the skin are destroyed and deeper skin layers are raw or charred. Any burns that cover an area larger than twice the size of the person's hand are considered third degree. *This is a medical emergency.*

Immediate treatment of third-degree burns consists of gently rinsing the area with clean, cool water, covering it with a sterile gauze or clean linen, and transporting the person to the nearest medical facility. Pain, fear, loss of fluids, and accompanying damage can lead to shock and death. *Do not leave the person alone except to call for emergency help.* If the child is conscious, give plenty of fluids to drink. If another person is available, you might have him or her prepare the following drink, which helps prevent shock by replacing fluids and balancing the blood: To a quart of water add 1/2 teaspoon salt, 1/2 teaspoon baking soda, 2–3 tablespoons honey or sugar, and, if available, some lemon juice. Give sips as often as possible. This drink may also be given after emergency treatment.

Burns, especially severe ones, are very frightening. Since fear itself can cause the person to be more vulnerable to pain and shock, help him into a comfortable position, loosen his clothing, and help him relax with gentle touching and a calm voice. Bach Rescue Remedy, a Bach flower remedy, 4 drops given every five minutes, relieves fear and shock.

Homeopathic arnica 30x can also be given every five minutes as needed. Other pain-relief and nerve-calming remedies include valerian tincture, skullcap tincture, and chamomile tea.

Those who have been severely burned need to continue drinking plenty of fluids throughout the healing process and should eat a high-protein diet along with plenty of fresh vegetables. Vitamins A, E, and C and zinc are particularly recommended for healing burns. After the burn has begun to heal, vitamin E oil may be applied regularly to the area to minimize scarring.

❖ CAR SICKNESS ❖

While not an illness, car sickness is very unpleasant for the affected passenger (and potentially for everyone in the car!). As a child, I had lots of experience with those sensations of head-swimming nausea. I hope these remedies and tips make your child's travels more pleasant.

GENERAL RECOMMENDATIONS

- Keep a window slightly open (even just a "crack" will do) so that your child will get some fresh air. This is a big help. Don't smoke in the car, and keep the heat at a moderate setting to avoid stuffiness.
- Let your child loosen his coat, any collar around his neck, his belt, and even open the top button of his pants to relieve any feelings of restriction. Wearing a seat belt is an important safety practice but may also contribute to car sickness, so make frequent stops on long trips so the child can unbuckle and get out of the car to walk around.
- Discourage the child from reading in the car because it often leads to queasiness. A small portable tape deck and some story tapes are a good replacement and an effective distraction from the nausea.
- If you'll be eating in the car, avoid sweet and oily foods. Focus on light snacks and meals such as vegetable sticks and dips, whole-grain pretzels, and simple sandwiches with cheese or other protein. Keep plenty of these foods available for snacks. Carbonated water also settles the stomach, so have that for a beverage.

HERBAL REMEDIES

- Ginger candies or tea can be used as needed to allay nausea. To prepare the tea, steep 1 teaspoon of finely grated fresh ginger root in 1 cup boiling water for twenty minutes. Strain and sweeten. (You can carry this delicious tea in a thermos.) Look for the candies at a local health-food store.

- Peppermint candies also prevent and relieve car sickness. Give your child a few drops of valerian tincture before the candy if car sickness is a big problem. This can be repeated as necessary, but the number of drops given over the course of a day should not exceed one-half of your child's weight. Also, do not use for more than a week at a time.
- Umeboshi (sour plum) candies are a nice change of taste, a delicious combination of sweet and sour, and they're great for all kinds of queasiness.
- Calm Child Formula, developed by herbalist Michael Tierra, is a wonderful nervine and digestive calmer, helping to allay the sickness and bringing the child a sense of tranquility. It can be used as a tonic, making it especially helpful on long car trips. It can be purchased in tincture form under the "Planetary Formulas" label, or it can be prepared at home as an infusion or syrup. The recipe calls for 2 parts each of catnip, chamomile, lemon balm, and valerian root, and 1 part each of lady's slipper and hawthorn berries.
- A couple of charcoal tablets can quickly absorb stomach acidity, decreasing nausea and headaches. These are a must for your first-aid travel kit. They are nearly miraculous for easing indigestion, mild dysentery, nausea, and related headaches.
- Sandalwood is FOR EXTERNAL USE ONLY! However, the scent of sandalwood oil is exceptionally settling to the nerves and the stomach. Rub a few drops onto your child's wrist like perfume, and he can smell it when he feels "woozy."

❖ CHICKENPOX ❖

Most children develop a reaction to the chickenpox virus (varicella) about ten to twenty-one days after exposure. Initial symptoms are a slight fever, mild cold symptoms, possible fatigue, and loss of appetite; in some instances there are no symptoms. One or two days later the typical chickenpox rash develops. It starts as red dots, often on the upper body, which soon turn into fluid-filled dots over red bases. These open and then are crusted over with very itchy scabs. New pox can continue to form for a few days. Some children develop only a mild case while others may have hundreds of spots. The virus is contagious until all of the spots have crusted over. One bout of chickenpox generally confers lifelong immunity. Some adults, however, develop shingles, which are caused by the same virus.

While this illness is uncomfortable because of the scabs' itchiness and the general cold symptoms, it is serious only if the pox become infected or in the rare event that any pox develop in the eyes. For chickenpox in the eyes, seek medical care.

To treat infected pox, follow the internal and external remedies under "Abscesses."

REMEDIES FOR CHICKENPOX

The natural treatment of chickenpox aims at helping your child discharge the illness with a minimum of discomfort, relaxing the nerves so the child can rest, providing relief from itching, and promoting healing of the skin.

- The severity of chickenpox may be influenced by the foods your child eats. Diets heavy in processed foods and even too many rich natural foods aggravate many skin rashes. A simple and wholesome diet will go a long way toward preventing and minimizing illness.
- Treat the initial cold symptoms described in "Colds."
- The following herbal combination, in infusion or tincture, acts as a blood purifier, helping to relieve the infection and reduce the rash. Mix the following dried herbs (or use the tinctures): 1/2 ounce echinacea root, or 20 drops tincture; 1/4 ounce burdock root, or 10 drops tincture; 1/4 ounce calendula blossoms, or 10 drops tincture; 1 tablespoon peppermint leaves (omit if using tinctures).

    Steep 1 ounce per quart of boiling water for four hours. Take by the mouthful throughout the day. If using tinctures, take in 1/4 cup warm water four times daily.
- Give 5 to 15 drops of skullcap tincture as needed or any of the calming teas such as Mother's Milk Tea II (see "Colic [or the Sunset Blues]" in Chapter 7) or Calm Child Formula (see "Car Sickness" in this chapter) to reduce irritability and discomfort.
- As much as possible, keep your child from scratching the pox to prevent scarring and infection. If necessary, provide your child with cotton gloves; put thin socks over babies' hands to keep them from scratching.
- Any of the following baths will reduce irritation, inflammation, and itching:

Burdock root and comfrey root bath: Make an infusion using 2 ounces of each herb per half gallon of water. Add to a warm bath, and let your child play in it as long as she likes.

Oatmeal bath: Fill a large cotton sock halfway with dry rolled oats, and tie the top closed with a rubber band or string. Fill your tub to the desired level with warm water, and put the sock and your child in the tub. You or your child can squeeze the sock in the water until it starts to exude oat milk. The sock should then be rubbed all over your child, and he should soak in the milky water. Oats are an emollient and an excellent remedy for many irritated skin conditions. (To clean the sock, empty it by turning it inside out and then launder as usual.)

Baking soda bath: Baking soda is another oldtime remedy for chickenpox and itchy skin irritations. If it is all you have on hand, it will serve quite well. Simply sprinkle 1/2 cup baking soda under the faucet while running the bathwater, and let your child soak.

Baths may be taken several times a day. Use fresh ingredients each time.

- After the bath, you can apply calendula, chickweed, or plantain in salve, ointment, or oil form. The following ingredients make an excellent healing salve: 1/4 ounce each of calendula blossoms, chickweed, plantain, comfrey leaves, and chamomile flowers; 1 tablespoon echinacea tincture; 1 cup olive oil; and 4 to 6 tablespoons grated beeswax. See "Herbal Preparations" in Chapter 4 for directions on how to make salves.
- Slippery elm powder can be sprinkled onto sores that are wet, oozy, or slow to scab over. It will quell the itching and dry the fluids, allowing the sores to crust over and heal.

❖ Chills ❖

Chills commonly occur after exposure to wet and cold conditions and may lower the resistance enough to allow illness to take hold. If your child has become chilled, warming him could allay sickness. Give your child a warm herbal bath with rosemary, chamomile, thyme, or lavender infusions. Dry him thoroughly, and dress him in warm clothing. (You may even want to have him put on a hat because so much heat is lost through the head.) Then provide a cup of warm soup or tea and plenty of cuddling in the covers!

Chills also accompany fevers. The warming teas that follow can also be used during a fever. This may seem contradictory, but it is simple to understand. The teas increase the circulation and ease the surface tension of the body, causing the child to sweat while still bringing deep warmth to the body. Keep the child dry and covered because the evaporation of the sweat could bring on further chills.

Chronic chills are sometimes a sign of iron deficiency, so see the section on anemia to see if your child is exhibiting other symptoms of iron deficiency.

HERBAL RECOMMENDATIONS

Choose any of these flavorful beverages that you think your child will enjoy:

- *Garlic lemonade:* Finely mince 2 cloves fresh garlic and place in a 1-quart Mason jar. Fill the jar with boiling water and cover for thirty minutes. Strain out the garlic, and to the liquid add the juice of one whole lemon. Sweeten to taste with honey. Give as warm as possible, and offer as much as the child can drink.
- *Ginger tea:* Pour 1 cup boiling water over 1 teaspoon of fresh grated ginger root. Steep for twenty minutes, strain, sweeten, and drink hot. Repeat as often as desired. Add lemon for taste if the child likes it.
- *Warming broth:* This is particularly good for warming the hands and feet and for chills accompanying a cold. To prepare, chop one onion and mince two cloves of garlic and 1 tablespoon of fresh gingerroot. Sauté in 1 tablespoon olive or sesame oil for two to three minutes. Add 4 cups water and simmer for thirty minutes. To this add 1 tablespoon (or more to taste) of miso paste and stir until dissolved. Next dissolve 1 tablespoon kudzu root in 1/4 cup cold water. Add this to the broth, stirring constantly while you cook for another minute. Serve warm. You can give your child just the broth or some of the onions as well.

❖ CHOKING ❖

Methods to deal with choking are beyond the scope of herbal treatments and this book. However, I strongly encourage all parents to take a cardio-pulmonary resuscitation (CPR) class where you learn mouth-to-mouth resuscitation, CPR, and other techniques, such as the Heimlich maneuver, to help someone who is choking. A one-day inexpensive course (usually costing no more than twenty dollars) is available from the American Red Cross and the American Heart Association. It's a worthwhile investment.

Babies and young children will often instinctively spit out nonfood items. Nevertheless, it is best to keep small objects, like hard candies, raisins, nuts, chips, and pebbles out of their reach. Encouraging children to be calm when they eat and to chew their food well before swallowing will help prevent choking (and encourage healthy digestion). Teach children never to run with candy, gum, or any food in their mouths.

❖ Colds and Flu ❖

The word *cold* is a catchall term that describes symptoms such as runny nose, scratchy throat, stuffy head, achiness, headache, indigestion (nausea, stomach ache, vomiting, diarrhea), and fever. Most kids with healthy immune systems get over a cold within a week with nothing more than tender loving care. As the old doctors' joke goes, "a cold will go away in a week by itself and seven days with medicine."

Influenza (flu) is an acute respiratory infection with some or all of these symptoms: fever, severe achiness, sore throat, congestion, lack of appetite, and extreme lassitude. In the past, influenza was dreaded, sometimes reached epidemic proportions, and even now causes occasional fatalities, but this is usually in the very young, in the elderly, and in those already weakened by malnutrition or other causes, such as underlying heart disease or pulmonary disease. While influenza generally is not a serious disease and is treatable at home or with medical care, it can be really draining even for strong, healthy adults. Be prepared for kids to run high fevers and sleep a lot for a few days!

Colds and flu frequently are a reflection of a temporary dip in immunity that is most often caused by insufficient rest. Too many rich foods, stress, or exposure to cold and dampness can also precipitate an occurrence. Care aims at relieving your child's temporary discomforts and bolstering overall health. Frequent colds can make your child vulnerable to deeper respiratory infections. Untreated, flu can settle into the chest and bring about a secondary infection of pneumonia, so be diligent in your care. Early and consistent attention, along with adequate time for convalescence, should keep all colds and flu from becoming problematic.

General Recommendations

- The most important things you can do for your child when she has a cold are to (1) encourage lots of rest; (2) simplify her diet (include whole grains, vegetable soups, and locally available seasonal fruits); (3) give plenty of water, especially if fever is present; and (4) help her feel comfortable.

- If the child has no appetite, don't force him to eat but *do push fluids if he has a fever.* Most children will resume a hearty appetite after a day or so of skipping regular meals. A light diet enables their bodies to do the work of healing without taxing the diges-tion. Giving your child "treat" foods such as ice cream is not ben-eficial and will only aggravate the cold.

HERBAL RECOMMENDATIONS

- For specific symptoms, see those headings—for example, "Aches," "Coughs and Congestion," and "Fevers."
- Echinacea, either in infusion or tincture, can be given four times a day to bolster immunity and eliminate infection.
- Chamomile, lemon balm, and catnip are the most commonly used and gentlest remedies known for children's colds. They reduce tension in the body, relieve headache, stomach upsets, and rest-lessness; and, in addition, are pleasant tasting. They should be prepared as infusions, either alone or in combination, and can be drunk freely. Serve these teas warm; otherwise they cause fre-quent urination.
- Give 250 to 500 milligrams of vitamin C along with each dose of echinacea. It is known to reduce infections and prevent their recurrence.
- Garlic lemonade or garlic in any form, ginger tea (see "Chills"), or kudzu-apple juice may be used as a beverage to reduce cold symptoms, warm and strengthen the child, and increase resistance to illness. All can be given during the cold and as a regular part of the diet.

    Kudzu-apple juice is a favorite beverage remedy around our house. It is so delicious that our kids ask for it even when they are quite well. Kudzu is a vine of Japanese origin (sometimes consid-ered invasive) that grows in the southeastern United States. The root yields a white starch similar to arrowroot but more nutritious and medicinal. It is known in Eastern medicine for relieving chills, aches, indigestion, and other symptoms of colds.

    To prepare, heat 3/4 cup unfiltered apple juice in a saucepan until it begins to simmer. Dissolve 1 tablespoon kudzu root into 1/4 cup cold apple juice. Stir this into the saucepan, and continue to stir until it comes to a boil. Reduce the temperature to low, and stir continuously for two to three minutes more. Cool until drinkable and then enjoy. The juice can be used as the child's main nourishment for a day. You can use pear juice in place of apple juice. A pinch of cinnamon can be added to either if the child has severe chills or diarrhea.

❖ CONJUNCTIVITIS (PINKEYE) ❖

Pinkeye is a highly contagious infection that affects the "conjunctiva"— the inner lining of the eyelids and the outer lining of the eyeballs. It is characterized by a sticky, yellow-green, itchy discharge that crusts over the eyelids, sometimes "gluing" them shut. This most commonly happens in the morning after the accumulated discharge from the night has thickened and hardened. A feeling like that of sand irritating the eyes causes a frequent urge to rub the eyes.

Pinkeye is not dangerous, but it is very uncomfortable, can be persistent, and is highly contagious. A few days of consistent and thorough treatment usually clears it up completely.

GENERAL RECOMMENDATIONS

- Encourage the child not to rub his eyes. This will cut down on the inflammation.
- Insist on frequent hand washing to prevent the infection from spreading to other family members (adults are not immune), as it is inevitable that the child will occasionally touch his eyes.
- Each family member with pinkeye should have his or her own personal towel to avoid spreading the infection around to everyone. Similarly, don't share pillows until after the infection is gone. Wash towels and pillowcases daily.
- Eliminate dairy foods, eggs, and flour products from the diet for the duration of the infection. These foods seem to encourage the production of the discharge.
- Offer plenty of water to drink.
- Breast milk is rich in antibodies that reduce many infections. If you are still lactating, a half teaspoon of your milk can be placed in the infected eyes of a child of any age. Repeat four times each day.

    Note: HIV can be transmitted through breast milk, even through the eyes. It is therefore best not to use breast milk other than your own.

HERBAL RECOMMENDATIONS

Choose one or more of the following suggestions. If only one eye is affected, you can apply the remedies only to that one or to both. To apply remedies to the eyes, tilt the child's head back or have her lie on your lap and place the drops in the inner corner of the eye. Let the liquid run outward toward the ear rather than toward the other eye. This will prevent the infection from contaminating the uninfected eye if only one eye is involved. The excess liquid can be patted dry with tissue paper, gauze, or a cloth (use a clean piece each time). Use a different piece to clean each eye. Do not place anything that has touched the eyes back into your remedy.

- Echinacea tincture should be given internally to boost the immune system. Give 1 drop per 5 pounds of body weight, four times a day. A red clover, burdock root, and chickweed tea may also be taken internally to help eliminate infection. Dose is 1/2 cup four times a day.
- Chamomile and goldenseal tea is a soothing, cooling eye healer and refresher. Prepare the chamomile by steeping 1 tablespoon of the herb in 1/2 cup boiling hot-water for twenty minutes. To this add 1/4 teaspoon goldenseal powder and steep for ten minutes more. Strain twice to remove small particles, and rinse the eyes or apply compresses three to six times a day.
- Chickweed, whose name means "little star lady," can put the twinkle back into red, sore eyes. Make an infusion using one handful of fresh plant to each cup of water. Apply as for the previous remedies, and use poultices of the steeped plant materials directly on the eyes. Discard the material after each use.
- Eyebright is traditionally used for eye problems. Prepare a standard infusion and rinse the eyes or apply compresses.

WHEN TO SEEK MEDICAL CARE

If these treatments have not brought marked improvement in five days, or if the condition worsens after the treatment has begun, seek medical care. Signs of worsening include the infection spreading to the other eye, discomfort, vision difficulty, and increase in the quantity of discharge.

❖ CONSTIPATION ❖

Occasionally a child may become constipated—that is, go a day or two without having a bowel movement or have bowel movements requiring great effort. Stress, change in environment (like travel), dietary changes, lack of sleep, and illnesses can cause this condition. Children with otherwise regular bowel habits usually resolve a bout of constipation with little need for remedies.

Chronic constipation is often the result of stress, imbalanced diet, or both. It can be addressed herbally, but the emotional issues the child is dealing with (stress between parents or difficulty in school, for instance) must also be attended to and dietary changes must be made.

Regularity in eating, sleeping, and sitting on the toilet is probably the most important ingredient in helping your child eliminate every day. Rushing children through breakfast and then making them rush to school causes physical reactions that easily translate into constipation. Most adults drink a cup of coffee in the morning to get themselves "up and going"; and, in fact, coffee is a natural laxative. Unfortunately, it's also addictive, and using it sets an unhealthy example for our children. Rather than raising our kids to become dependent on coffee or laxatives, we can teach them healthy habits that encourage and preserve natural body functions.

Allow children to take their time in the morning, and avoid confrontations and commands that cause them to feel small, withdrawn, or pressured. Warm cereals such as oatmeal and cream of rice are natural laxatives. The addition of raisins during cooking enhances the effect. Bran muffins made with molasses and raisins are also laxatives. Each of these foods is nutritious as well.

Teach your child to take a few minutes to sit on the toilet before he leaves for school. He can be taught to consciously relax his muscles. Often, just making this a habit at a similar time each day is a remedy in itself. This is really important because many kids who feel the need to go when they get to school just hold it until they get home, leading to further constipation as well as autointoxication (self-poisoning) from reabsorbed materials that were meant to be eliminated.

You may want to try putting a low stool under the child's feet while he sits on the toilet. A more physiologically correct position for elimination, it prevents straining and can help prevent hemorrhoids later in life. In fact, most people around the world who have no modern conveniences use a squatting position for elimination.

Dietary Recommendations

- Children prefer foods that are starchy and fatty like bread, pasta, crackers, cheese, butter, and peanut butter. These foods seem to provide the calories they need for growing and being active, but it is important that they be made from whole grains or from natural sources with minimal processing. In addition, provide a variety of fresh produce daily. Because a diet with adequate fiber will prevent constipation and lack of essential nutrients such as iron can cause it, a whole-foods diet with herbal supplementation will help your child meet his nutritional needs and prevent a variety of health problems.

- Children should be encouraged to drink plenty of water, at least four glasses a day. A cup of warm water each morning will encourage bowel movements.
- Include stewed and soaked dried fruits (figs, prunes, and raisins), stewed apples, and molasses in your child's diet.
- If your child is experiencing constipation, decrease as much as possible the amount of dairy foods, meat, eggs, wheat, and nut butters that your child eats until the problem is resolved.

HERBAL RECOMMENDATIONS

Any or all of the following remedies may be incorporated into your child's diet as they are all nutritive and many are delicious. These herbs provide bulk to the colon and gently stimulate digestion. Other herbs not included here are stronger acting on the bowels (senna and rhubarb, for example), but gentle remedies are preferable; they cause no griping or pain and do not result in dependence.

- *Smooth-Move infusion:* Make an infusion of the following herbs in 1 pint of water: 2 teaspoons slippery elm powder, 1 teaspoon fennel seeds, 1 teaspoon licorice root, 1/4 teaspoon ginger root (powdered). Steep for one hour and strain. Dosage is 1 tablespoon to children under two years, 1/4 cup to children ages two to seven, and 1/2 to 1 cup for older children. The infusion can be given as needed until the child has had a bowel movement.

  Slippery elm provides the bulk and moisture that aids elimination while the remaining herbs ease gas to prevent possible cramping. Fennel and licorice are also mildly laxative.
- Mix 1 teaspoon of slippery elm powder per 1 cup of warm apple juice. Stir well. Give as much as the child will take. This is great for children of all ages but particularly for babies.
- Flax seed, psyllium, and carob powder are bulk laxatives that can be used in drinks, sprinkled onto foods, or made into treats for kids. Plantain seeds can substitute for flax seeds. They grow abundantly in many regions and are free if you are willing to take the time to harvest them. Here are some recipes:

  Fruit balls: Rich in nutrients, fruit balls are a healthy treat for kids of all ages and a great laxative. They are real sticky so get kids to brush teeth after eating them to prevent cavities. To make them, first slowly grind 1/2 cup raisins, 1/2 cup prunes, 1/2 cup almonds, and 1/4 cup flax seeds in a blender or food processor.

Add a little water as needed to form a slightly sticky dough. Form into 2-inch balls and roll in shredded coconut or almond meal. Have fun creating your own variations.

Carob smoothie: This recipe was inspired by Humbart Santillo's book *Natural Healing with Herbs* (see "Further Reading"). He calls it a "good morning drink." Mix 1 teaspoon powdered flax seed, 1 teaspoon hulled sesame seeds, 1 tablespoon unroasted carob powder, and 1 teaspoon honey. Mix in a blender with 1 cup warm water or soy milk. One to 2 cups of this beverage usually promotes a quick response.

- Yellow dock and dandelion syrup, or tinctures of these herbs, are a reliable remedy for chronic constipation. These herbs encourage bowel movements, stimulate the liver, and nourish the blood. The syrup is recommended here for children over three years but can be used in smaller dosages by younger children. The syrup is more nutritive, but the tinctures are also effective. Dosage for the tinctures is 15 to 30 drops of each in water twice daily.

  To prepare the syrup, steep 1 ounce each of the herbs in 1 pint boiling water for eight hours. Strain; then simmer uncovered over low heat until only 1 cup of liquid remains. Sweeten with 1/4 cup of either honey or molasses, cool to room temperature, and then cover and store in the fridge for up to two months. Dose is 2 teaspoons daily for children under seven years, 2 tablespoons daily for those older. In addition to remedying constipation, this formula is a primary treatment for anemia.

OTHER RECOMMENDATIONS

- Massage your child's abdomen clockwise in a big circle, starting just above the pubic bone (at "six o'clock"). When you come down the final part of the circle, exert firm downward pressure without being rough. Imagine your hands easing blockages and relaxing tensions in the child's stomach. You can use a little oil on your hands, which you should rub in your palms before placing them on the child's tummy. Chamomile, lavender, and rose oils are excellent choices. Teach your child to visualize his abdominal and pelvic muscles as relaxed and comfortable. Many people store tension in this area, and it is never too early to learn to relax there. For chronic constipation, do this about three times per week at bedtime, and teach your child to massage his or her abdomen upon awakening.
- Plenty of exercise in the fresh air will keep the bowels healthy. If your child sits in school most of the day, then comes home and

watches television and does homework, she may not be getting enough physical exercise. Turn off the tube and have her go outside to play, run, ride a bicycle, jump rope. An after-dinner walk is a wonderful family tradition. Not only does adequate exercise prevent bowel problems, but it also enhances overall digestion and assimilation of nutrients as well as circulation. When children get enough exercise and fresh air, they also have an easier time concentrating on their work and sleeping at night.

❖ COUGHS AND CONGESTION ❖

The causes of coughs and congestion are highly variable: exposure to cold air or dry heat, allergens (dust, pollen, mold), bacterial or viral infection, stress or fatigue, or dietary factors, such as overconsumption of dairy products. Generally speaking, a cough is the body's way of trying to expel or eliminate something from the breathing passages. Because herbalism seeks to cure the causes of illness rather than just treat symptoms, curing a cough means determining and addressing its cause.

In addition to their sources, coughs can have different qualities: wet, dry, productive, irritable, mild, and harsh, to name a few. You therefore need to do some detective work and learn the most appropriate restoratives for your child. The following section will help you to do this.

WHEN TO SEEK MEDICAL CARE

Persistent or severe coughs, especially if accompanied by breathing difficulty, increased breathing rate, blueness of the skin, blood in the mucus, or loss of weight, or coughs lasting longer than two weeks require prompt medical attention.

GENERAL RECOMMENDATIONS

- Follow the dietary recommendations in "Colds and Flu," providing plenty of soft and liquid foods that don't aggravate the coughing. While children may crave cold foods or beverages, provide only room-temperature and warm victuals.
- Massage is an excellent way to help your child relax if the cough is disturbing sleep. For specific massage techniques, see "Asthma." For general massage, use your intuition and rub your child's feet or back slowly and deeply to promote rest. Avoid tickling. See "Further Reading" for recommended massage books.
- Visualization and progressive relaxation are also wonderful techniques to use in conjunction with massage or alone. Older

children can be taught to use these methods on their own. Again, see "Asthma" for a sample visualization and "Further Reading" for relevant books.

- During cold weather, when the heat is going and the air is dry, a good humidifier can go a long way to preventing a dry cough. I personally prefer to use warm (not cold) water in the humidifier, but this seems to be a matter of personal opinion. Add a couple drops of eucalyptus oil to the water to freshen the air.

HERBAL RECOMMENDATIONS

Herbs relieve coughs in a variety of ways. Some herbs function as expectorants, aiding in the bringing up and elimination of mucus. Examples of expectorants include anise seed, mullein, coltsfoot, elecampane, horehound, angelica, and lobelia. Expectorants can function as respiratory stimulants or relaxants, either by encouraging the loosening of mucus and stimulating the reflexes of the body to cough it up effectively, or by helping the muscles relax, allowing the child to clear mucus without spasmodic and irritable coughing.

Respiratory relaxants do exactly that: They relax the child enough to allow the easier elimination of mucus. Easing the cough also allows irritated mucus membranes in the respiratory passages to heal, reducing the severity and frequency of the coughing that is occurring as a result of irritation and inflammation. Almost any relaxing herbs can be beneficial to a child who has an irritable cough, but some are specifically for use during coughs. These include, to name a few, mullein, wild cherry bark, anise seed, licorice, lobelia, red clover blossoms, and angelica.

Demulcents are another category of herbs used to treat lung afflictions. These herbs, which may possess some of the previously mentioned qualities as well, tend to produce mucilaginous substances when combined with water. These substances have soothing, anti-inflammatory qualities, which are especially helpful for coughs due to irritation in the bronchial passages and throat. Demulcents have a moistening quality and so are particularly beneficial for dry throats and coughs. They include marshmallow root, comfrey root, slippery elm bark, violet leaves, flax seeds, and licorice root. Burdock root, chickweed, astragalus, and echinacea are not demulcents but have anti-inflammatory qualities and can enhance a cough remedy.

- To prepare your own personalized cough remedy, one specific to your child's needs, you can simply determine the type of cough your child seems to have and create a mixture with the appropriate herbs. For example, if the cough is very dry, emphasize demulcents; if the child seems to have a lot of mucus but is unable to clear it, expectorants are in order; and if the cough is of the irritable tickling type, perhaps relaxants are the most suitable choice. Combine at least one herb from each category, trying various combinations for taste. If you hit on a blend you really like, you can keep it on hand or turn it into a syrup that can keep refrigerated for months (see "Herbal Preparations" in Chapter 4).

- A cough syrup blend that I find effective and pleasant for use with children consists of 3 grams each of comfrey root, coltsfoot, mullein leaves, marshmallow root, licorice root, thyme, and anise seeds; 1 1/2 grams each of wild cherry bark and burdock root; and 1/2 gram each of slippery elm bark and lobelia. Sometimes I add up to 3 grams of either violet leaves or red clover blossoms. Mix all the herbs and steep in 1 quart boiling water for two hours. Strain the liquid into a pot and simmer gently until it is reduced to 1 cup of liquid (discard the plant material). Sweeten with 1/4 cup honey (for children under one year, omit the honey and replace with maple syrup or sugar to taste). After the syrup cools to room temperature, store it in a jar in the fridge. It will keep for months. Dosage is 1 teaspoon as needed for children one to three years old, 1 tablespoon as needed for older children, and 2 tablespoons as needed for adults. (*Note:* This blend is not for use by pregnant women.)

- Babies and children alike benefit from herbal baths that relax the breathing and loosen congestion. Add 1 to 5 drops of eucalyptus, thyme, or wintergreen oil to a warm bath, or alternatively, use a strong infusion of thyme (steep 1 ounce of the herb in a quart of hot water for thirty minutes, strain, and add to the bathwater).

- For babies and young children prepare kudzu-apple juice (see "Colds and Flu") or slippery elm drink. To prepare the latter, stir 1 teaspoon of slippery elm powder into either warm apple juice or warm water sweetened with a bit of maple syrup. Both are delicious. These drinks can be used as beverages and given to baby by cup, spoon, or even medicine dropper.

- Another fun way to use slippery elm for coughs is to prepare lozenges, or as my kids call them, "Slippery Elm Balls." Mix a couple tablespoons of slippery elm powder in a bowl with enough honey to make a dough. You can even add a few drops of flavoring such as lemon, mint, or vanilla. Roll the dough into a long, thin "snake" (remember kindergarten?); then slice the roll into quarter-inch pieces. They can be eaten as is or rolled in a bit of the powder and set aside to dry until slightly hard. Kids can suck them as often as they want.

- For acute coughs associated with colds and respiratory infections, garlic-lemonade is indispensable. It soothes a cough, has antiviral and antibacterial properties, strengthens the immune system, and aids in expectoration. Steep four to six cloves of garlic in 1 quart boiling water for thirty minutes, strain, and add lemon and honey to taste. Serve hot and often. Ginger tea (see "Chills") with lemon and honey has similar properties and can be used alternately for variety.

- Also useful is a Chinese herbal preparation called "loquat syrup." Often available at natural-food stores and at Chinese herbal pharmacies (visit the Chinatown in your city), it is a thick mentholated syrup that is pleasant to take and quiets the cough.

- In addition to cough remedies, if there is infection, give echinacea tincture, 10 to 35 drops (the younger the child the lower the dosage), and 250 milligrams of vitamin C four times a day. This will prevent the infection from worsening and offset secondary problems such as ear infection, which often occurs with upper respiratory congestion. If the child is old enough to swallow them give garlic perles, or be sure to give garlic lemonade.

- A good old home remedy for coughs is 1 part each of brandy, lemon, and honey. Dosage is 1 teaspoon as needed, but not, of course, to the point of drunkenness. This is a good bedtime cough remedy for kids because it promotes sleep. You can periodically add *one drop* of either thyme or eucalyptus oil to the teaspoon, *but no more than 4 drops per day.*

- For persistent coughs or bronchitis, in addition to the above remedies, you can use a mustard plaster to bring warmth and circulation to the chest area, which reduces coughing and speeds healing. *Do not use a mustard plaster on children under three years, anyone who is asleep or unconscious, or anyone who, for whatever reason, is unable to communicate with you if the plaster becomes uncomfortable.* Mustard can be caustic, so improper application can cause severe skin burns. The process may seem elaborate or complicated, but after doing it once it will be simple. Carefully read through the directions before beginning.

HOW TO MAKE A MUSTARD PLASTER

Supplies needed: 1/4 cup dried mustard powder; two cotton kitchen tow-els; one large bath towel; hot water; a large bowl; a warm, wet wash cloth; some salve or petroleum jelly.

Instructions:

1. Lay out one kitchen towel on a flat surface. Spread the mustard pow-der onto the towel, leaving a 1-inch border around the edge uncovered. Next, fold the bottom border upward over the edge of the powder. This will keep the powder from falling out. Place the second towel over the first one, and starting from each of the short edges, roll the edges to the center, like a scroll.

2. Place the scroll into the bowl and cover with very hot water. Bring the bowl and all the other supplies into your child's room. Be certain there are no drafts in the room.

3. Place the large bath towel open on a pillow, take off the child's shirt, and liberally spread the salve or petroleum jelly onto the nipples to protect them from getting blistered or burned. They are more sensitive than the skin.

4. Thoroughly wring the water out of the mustard-filled towel when it is cool enough to be handled. Open the mustard bandage with the pow-der side up, and place the mustard-covered side against the child's chest and as far around the back as it will reach. The child should quickly lay back on the bath towel, which you then wrap over the plaster. Cover the child with blankets.

5. To prevent burns, remove the plaster immediately when the child says it feels hot or is stinging. This may be after only a few minutes. After removing the plaster, wash the area with the damp wash cloth and cover the child with blankets to prevent chill. Never leave the plaster on a child under the age of eight for more than five minutes. Adults can tolerate it for a maximum of 20 minutes. Do not repeat more than twice a day for two days, and discontinue if the area is be-coming red. Never leave the child unattended while the plaster is on.

With some of the remedies described above, you will find that you are able to minimize the discomfort of a cough, shorten a cough's dura-tion, and perhaps learn to prevent respiratory infections from occurring with any frequency in your home.

❖ CUTS, SCRAPES, AND WOUNDS ❖

A healthy child is unlikely to experience a major infection from a minor injury, so you can usually care for minor scrapes and small cuts simply by washing them thoroughly under running water to clean out all particles of dirt. You can then wash the area with an infusion (1 ounce herb to 1 pint water) or a dilute tincture (1 dropperful to 1/4 cup water) of any of these herbs: calendula, echinacea, rosemary, goldenseal, lavender, thyme, or chaparral. Alternatively, you can apply diluted apple cider vinegar (1/4 to 1 cup water) as a rinse. All of these have antimicrobial properties and thus reduce bacteria and the chances of infection. If you don't have any of these ingredients at home, you can use hydrogen peroxide. In any case, water is the most important element. After the cut scabs over, you can apply healing salve to reduce itching and scarring.

Deep cuts need more care but often can be treated at home if you are attentive. Most cuts bleed profusely, making the situation appear more serious than it is. A small amount of bleeding is actually desirable because it cleans the wound from the inside out. To stop excessive bleeding, apply firm pressure to the wound (you can use a clean cloth to cover the wound as you do this) for a few minutes or until the bleeding stops.

WHEN TO SEEK MEDICAL CARE

If a cut is spurting blood, a major blood vessel may have been severed. THIS IS A MEDICAL EMERGENCY. Apply pressure with a clean towel to slow the bleeding, and transport the child to medical care immediately! If stitches are called for, they must be done within eight hours of the injury to be effective and to prevent infection. If the injury is deep, is made by a dirty object, or occurred near any areas that are high in risk for tetanus (near farm animals, pastures, or stables, for example), or if a puncture wound has not bled, quickly get your child a tetanus shot if he or she is not currently vaccinated.

If blood is flowing steadily but the damage does not seem extensive, briefly run water over the injury site to clean it out and to be able to inspect it. Water will usually slow down the bleeding. If not, you can put pressure on the area with a clean towel or gauze.

Many cuts heal well with minimal scarring even without stitches. A good rule of thumb is to see whether the sides of the cut match up on their own. If they do, stitches usually can be avoided. If they don't, you may wish to try "butterfly bandages," specially shaped bandages that work like stitches and are available at pharmacies.

If your child is currently vaccinated for tetanus, call your physician to see whether a booster shot is needed. To prevent tetanus, wash cuts very well under running water. Never put oily substances (such as salve) over a cut since it may seal in the bacteria. Tetanus can thrive only in an anaerobic (nonoxygenated) environment, so using hydrogen peroxide is advisable because it oxygenates the cut. Allow the cut to bleed moderately to clean itself out. Where tetanus is a concern, check it out.

It is fine to wash the wound with tapwater initially. Deep cuts should then be thoroughly washed with boiled water or sterile saline every few hours. You can use any of the herbs mentioned at the beginning of this section as well. Echinacea tincture can be taken internally, 1 drop for every 2 pounds of body weight four times a day, to prevent infections.

❖ DIARRHEA ❖

Diarrhea is the frequent passage of watery stools. It can be the result of an intestinal inflammation, virus or bacteria, stress or emotional upset, dietary changes, teething, or general illness (such as a cold). It is the body's natural mechanism for eliminating illness from the body and in this sense is a desirable response. A child can also have digestive weakness that leads to chronic diarrhea. In such a case, prevent dehydration by providing the child with plenty of fluids. Diarrhea may persist for a few days, but as long as the child is otherwise healthy and is able to consume fluids, it is okay to let it run its course.

WHEN TO SEEK MEDICAL CARE

The danger of diarrhea is that it can lead to dehydration, which can develop into a life-threatening condition. The symptoms of dehydration include dry mouth (you should feel moisture when you touch your child's tongue), a warm, dry feeling to the skin; rapid pulse; low fever; and very little urination. If a child is severely dehydrated, when you pinch a little of his skin between your fingers, the skin will not quickly return to its original flat shape but will remain slightly tented. If you suspect your child is *becoming* dehydrated and cannot get the child to take or retain fluids, seek immediate medical help. Of course, any child complaining of unusual symptoms, such as extreme abdominal pain and tenderness, needs further attention.

General Recommendations

- The most important thing to do for a child with diarrhea is to give fluids frequently. A child seven years or older can drink about a cup of liquid every hour; give fluids by the quarter cup every fifteen to twenty minutes. Give slightly less to younger children and slightly more to older children. The point is to keep as much liquid going in as is coming out. Room-temperature or slightly warm water, broth, and herbal infusions are the best choices. It is preferable not to give soft drinks or other heavily sugared or processed beverages, but you need to get fluids into the child, so use your discretion and common sense.
- Eating a lot of fruits, juices, and cold foods such as ice cream can result in diarrhea so avoiding overconsumption of these foods, especially during the colder months of the year, reduces its likelihood. An allergic reaction to a food also can cause diarrhea. If your child has diarrhea regularly, look for a correlation between diet and a recurrence. Once you isolate the probable allergen, you can experiment by removing that food from the diet and see if the problem returns. Many children eventually outgrow food allergies, so you can try the food again at a later time.
- If the child has loose bowel movements, provide foods that are easy to digest, warming, and nourishing. Soups, cream of rice, and cream of wheat are excellent for regulating the bowels.
- Diarrhea is uncomfortable, so do your best to involve your child in enjoyable activities.
- Diarrhea often causes extreme anal irritation. You can gently put salve around the anus to alleviate the problem. If the buttocks or surrounding areas become irritated, you can use healing salve, calendula oil, aloe vera gel, or slippery elm powder.
- A hot salt pack can be excellent for allaying diarrhea. It warms the intestines, reducing cramping and adding the tonification sometimes needed to reduce diarrhea. Directions for preparing and using salt packs can be found under "Vomiting."

Herbal Recommendations

- The most widely used remedies are infusions of blackberry root and red raspberry leaf, both of which are astringent and help tonify the intestinal mucus membranes. For an effective formula to treat both acute and chronic diarrhea as well as intestinal weakness, mix 1 tablespoon each of the following herbs and prepare an infusion in 1 pint of water: blackberry root, slippery elm bark (whole, not powdered if possible), comfrey root, and red raspberry leaves. If the child has a lot of cramping or a cold feeling in the abdomen, add 1 teaspoon fresh ginger root or 1/2 teaspoon dried. Steep for two hours, or simmer for twenty minutes and then strain. Give 2 teaspoons to 4 tablespoons depending on the child's age, and repeat every one to four hours, as needed.

Comfrey and slippery elm lend soothing qualities to irritated intestines and calm digestion, naturally helping to reduce diarrhea.

- *Cinnamon tea:* Cinnamon warms the intestines and lower body, easing cramping and reducing diarrhea that results from excessive exposure to cold or consumption of cold foods. Steep 1 teaspoon of cinnamon powder in 1 cup of boiling water for twenty minutes. Sweeten with honey and add milk if desired. Give by the tablespoon as needed. Do not give to children under one year of age.

For a child of any age, sprinkle cinnamon onto applesauce for a delicious snack. A folk remedy for loose stools because of the pectin in the fruit, applesauce helps solidify bowel movements.

❖ DYSENTERY ❖

Dysentery is an infection caused by organisms such as bacteria or amoebas and is usually contracted from ingesting contaminated food or water. Symptoms include diarrhea, foul-smelling gas, cramping, and, often, vomiting. If you have any question about the safety of a water source such as a stream, don't drink from it, or, if you must, boil the water first. Even rinsing your mouth or brushing your teeth with contaminated water can lead to a full-blown case of dysentery. While dysentery is not very common in modern cities that have adequate plumbing and sanitation, families who go hiking or drink from springs or wells may encounter it.

WHEN TO SEEK MEDICAL CARE

Refer to the warning signs for diarrhea and vomiting. As with those conditions, your greatest risk is dehydration.

HERBAL RECOMMENDATIONS

Follow the recommendations in "Vomiting" and "Diarrhea," along with the addition of these herbs:

- Give 1 drop of echinacea tincture per 2 pounds of the child's body weight, two to three times daily, plus 1 drop of goldenseal tincture per 5 pounds of body weight two to three times daily.

- Also give one to two tablets or capsules of activated charcoal powder three times daily.

Improvement should be noticeable within twenty-four hours of beginning treatment.

❖ EARACHES AND EAR INFECTIONS ❖

Localized pain and general irritability characterize middle-ear infections. Fever, swelling of the glands in the area, and hearing difficulty from the fluid in the ears may accompany the infection. Younger children often pull on their ears and may scream or cry suddenly and unexpectedly; older children will let you know about their extremely painful condition. Occasionally, a child can have fluid congestion and mild inflammation that causes hearing difficulties without the other symptoms of ear infection. If your child is having hearing difficulties, you can confirm it with an otoscope if you have one. If you see cloudiness, fluid, or a yellowish color (from pus), fluid reducing sound conduction in the ear is most likely causing your child's hearing difficulty. Follow the general and dietary recommendations listed below to reduce congestion and improve hearing.

Ear infections are the most prevalent complaint that land children in the doctor's office. They are almost completely preventable and easily remedied at home; yet they are one of the most common reasons that doctors prescribe antibiotics. While extreme chronic ear infections may lead to permanent hearing damage over time, an occasional infection rarely does so. Two physicians recently told me that even chronic ear congestion and inflammation can persist for many months or even for a couple of years without resulting in permanent hearing loss. Even rupture of the eardrum, which results from the pressure of fluid on the tympanic membrane, rarely causes hearing damage unless it occurs repeatedly. This is a far cry from the panic that is cast over most parents regarding their children's hearing when an ear infection occurs.

Redness of the visible parts of the ear and extreme tenderness when the ear lobe is touched or pulled characterize outer-ear inflammations and infections. This condition is commonly referred to as "swimmer's ear" because swimmers are prone to it from getting water in their ears. It can occur in others as well and is not dependent on swimming. Swimmers can prevent it by placing a couple of drops of rubbing alcohol or, even better, white vinegar in each ear after swimming to kill infectious organisms and dry the ear canal. It should be treated as other ear infections, because it can spread to the middle and inner ear.

Natural treatment of ear infections is, in the long run, more effective than antibiotics because it addresses the systemic and environmental roots of the problem in addition to dealing with the symptoms of pain and inflammation. Frequently, the child on antibiotics needs repeated cycles of progressively stronger medications because both the body and the strain of infection become resistant to the effects of the drugs. Antibiotics are meant for the treatment of bacterial infections; yet many ear infections are not the result of bacteria but of viruses. These organisms can only proliferate in an environment that supports their growth. The real treatment consists of strengthening the child and creating a healthy environment so he or she is not susceptible to the problem.

WHEN TO SEEK MEDICAL CARE

Earaches treated with natural remedies at the onset of the illness usually show rapid signs of improvement, often within just a few hours. Within twenty-four hours the severe discomfort and signs of infection should have passed. If your child is not responding to home care, if the infection rapidly seems worse, or if for any reason you suspect more than a simple ear infection, seek medical opinion. Ear infection can spread to the surrounding area, leading to serious complications. If the ear is draining, the eardrum may have ruptured. You may wish to see a physician to confirm this and to help you determine the best treatment.

GENERAL RECOMMENDATIONS

- As old fashioned as it might seem, a good wool hat goes a long way toward preventing head colds and ear infections. Wind can invade the body and quickly turn into an earache. Keep the head and ears well covered when the child goes out in cold or windy weather.
- Be conscious of your child's emotional environment. Is there something he or she "doesn't want to hear"? Time and time again, I have seen kids develop an earache in direct relationship to stress in their environments, particularly when their parents have been arguing. If this rings a bell for you, find peaceful ways to express yourselves to each other and to your children, and you will reduce the incidence of your child's earaches.
- A hot-water bottle wrapped in a towel (to avoid burning your child) can bring a lot of comfort to a painful ear. Used in conjunction with herbal eardrops, the heat is not only soothing but also brings healthy circulation to the area.
- Chinese remedial massage for children, known as "Tui Na," is extremely effective in combination with herbs. If your child has a

tendency to ear infections, I strongly urge you to purchase a copy of *Turtle Tails and Other Tender Mercies*, by Bob Flaws (see "Further Reading"). It is replete with directions for giving Tui Na for a variety of children's health conditions.

- You can give your child firm but gentle massage all around the jaw and head in the area adjacent to the ear. Massage in a downward direction behind the ear on the neck and apply gentle inward pressure in front of the ear toward the cheek (about where sideburns would be). This facilitates drainage of ear fluids and stimulates pressure points in the area. It may be uncomfortable to your child, so do it a few times a day for short periods.

DIETARY RECOMMENDATIONS

- Kids who drink a lot of juice and eat lots of fruit out of season, as well as those who eat a lot of dairy products and peanut butter, tend to get the most earaches. Cold-natured foods (foods that are cold in temperature and foods that cool the body down, such as those commonly eaten during summer or in tropical climates) and dairy products are prime culprits. They encourage the production of a lot of mucus in the upper respiratory system. The mucus can lead to congestion in the chest and ears, a ripe situation for an ear infection. Do not let your child have any juice or cold foods straight from the refrigerator until the infection has been gone for at least three days.

   If your child has a tendency toward earaches or general congestion, you may want to experiment with his or her diet and find alternatives (for example, herbal teas, local fruits in season, and warm snacks). Your goal is to promote warmth in the body and reduce mucus congestion. Some of the many macrobiotic cookbooks available can give you recipe ideas that will help you do this and still provide delicious and substantial meals. Most likely you will notice that your child has fewer recurrences, if any at all.

- Dairy products are up there on the list of foods that aggravate congestion. Congestion and colds frequently translate into ear infections. Limit your child's consumption of dairy foods, replacing them with other sources of calcium, minerals, and protein such as nuts, seeds, beans, leafy green vegetables, molasses, and occasionally very hard cheeses such as Parmesan or aged cheddar. Eventually your child is likely to outgrow the tendency to get earaches, and you may then resume dairy products in the diet. See "Further Reading" for books on nutrition and diet.

- Vitamin C in the form of a supplement is helpful for children with earaches, preventing infection from worsening and recurring. It gives the immune system a boost. Give 250 to 500 milligrams four times a day. Potatoes, leafy green vegetables, berries, broccoli, peppers, rose hips, cherries, and alfalfa sprouts are good food sources of vitamin C.

Herbal Recommendations

- The primary remedy for ear infections is garlic-mullein oil. Garlic is a natural antimicrobial, addressing infections of both a bacterial and viral nature. Mullein is an analgesic, relieving the pain associated with earaches.

  To prepare, place one whole bulb of finely chopped fresh garlic and 1 ounce of mullein flowers in a pint jar. Add olive oil until the jar is full. Stir with a chopstick or the handle of a wooden spoon to release air bubbles. Cover the jar and place in the sunlight for three weeks (two weeks in warm weather). Strain into a clean jar (discard plant material) and store in the refrigerator. It will keep for up to two years.

  If you need it in a hurry, a quicker method is to place all the above herbs and oil in a saucepan instead of a jar. Simmer over a *very low* flame (use a flame deflector if you have one) for thirty minutes. Strain, cool, and store as above.

  To use, place three to seven drops of the oil into the affected ear. The oil should be at room temperature or slightly warm. To warm it, put the drops in a spoon or a glass eyedropper and briefly hold a lit match to it. Test the oil against the underside of your wrist to make sure it is not too hot.

  Have the child rest with the affected ear up for five to ten minutes, keeping a warm hot-water bottle (covered with a towel) on the ear. After this time, let the child roll over and rest on the hot-water bottle for as long as it brings comfort. Repeat on the other ear if necessary. This can be repeated two or three times a day but may only be necessary once or twice as it is very effective.

- Calendula oil (which can be purchased or prepared the same way as the above oil) is also antiseptic and pain relieving. It can substitute for garlic-mullein oil and is used the same way.

- In addition to earache oils and vitamin C, the child should be given echinacea tincture to boost the immune system. Dosage is 1 drop per 2 pounds of body weight four times a day.

- Other herbs can also be used to help your child rest and minimize his or her discomfort. Chamomile makes an excellent tea and can also be made into an herbal pillow on which your child can sleep (see "Aches"). Skullcap tincture (15 drops) or valerian tincture (10 drops) can be given every couple of hours. Remember, if the pain is not going away or is getting worse, consult with someone with more experience. With the above care, however, this is unlikely.

- For a persistent ear infection, particularly if there is an outer-ear infection, place two to three drops of goldenseal tincture directly into the ear canal three to four times a day until it is completely cleared up.

- If persistent congestion is promoting ear infection, use a decongestant blend containing ephedra. Prepare a tea using 1 teaspoon each of ephedra, elder blossoms, and lemon balm. Steep for twenty minutes and serve 2 tablespoons four times a day to children under seven years, and 1/4 cup four times a day to children seven years and over. Elder is also a decongestant for the upper respiratory system, while lemon balm promotes rest and prevents digestive upsets from the use of elder. A decongestant tincture containing ephedra may be available at a natural-food store or herb shop. Follow dosage directions on the label.

    Warning: Excessive intake of ephedra can cause serious side effects. Before using this herb, refer to the directions in "Asthma" for specific guidelines.

❖ FEVERS ❖

Fever is not an illness. It is a process occurring as a response to and signal of illness. It is not the fever itself that needs to be eliminated. Rather, the task is to support and nourish the child while the body does the work of eliminating infection, regaining equilibrium, and healing.

Taken orally, normal temperature in a child is considered to be 98.6 degrees Fahrenheit, 97.6 degrees when taken under the armpit. Most kids over three are old enough to safely hold a thermometer in the mouth for three minutes. This gives an accurate reading unless the child has recently eaten or drunk something hot or cold. If so, wait fifteen minutes before checking. The pulse and breathing are likely to be more rapid than usual, and the child probably will want to sleep a lot. Fevers may occur in a variety of situations including infection, burns, heat stroke, or dehydration. Even exertion, exhaustion, and overexcitement can cause a child to run a slight fever. The particular cause of the fever should be determined and addressed. This section deals with fevers occurring with common ailments such as colds and flu or with no apparent illness, such as with teething or exhaustion.

If your child seems very ill, has a stiff neck (can't touch chin to chest without discomfort) or severe headache, has projectile vomiting (the vomit is coming out with considerable force), seems dazed or unresponsive, has sharp abdominal pains, or is rapidly getting worse despite your efforts, seek medical help immediately. Also, be aware of the signs of dehydration, including dry mucus membranes, sunken eyes, slipping in and out of consciousness, and tenting of the skin (see "Diarrhea"). Babies may exhibit a sunken soft spot on the head. All of these symptoms indicate an emergency.

The role of fever in illness is not completely understood, but prior to "modern medicine," traditional healers considered fever to be an innate fire motivated by the body's vital energy to heal the organism during illness or infection. During the past century, Western science has promoted the idea that fever itself is an illness and has sought to suppress it with aspirin, acetaminophen (Tylenol), and antibiotics. Current research on the human immune system is revealing that fever is not a disease but an immune system enhancer and stimulant. Fevers are now known to cause the production and release of chemicals in our bodies that actually combat infections. Increased temperature may also create an environment inhospitable to the growth of pathogenic organisms that in large populations in the body can lead to severe illness. What wise women, mothers, and traditional healers have known for ages, conventional medicine, still in its infancy, is just beginning to acknowledge. We may yet "discover" that it is the widespread suppression of the immune system that is contributing to the rise of autoimmune diseases.

Fever has another effect that often goes unnoticed. When children recover from a fever, they often demonstrate new skills and abilities. It is as if the heat of the fever served as a motivating developmental force. After a fever, a child frequently seems even stronger and healthier than before, as if impurities had been burned away, leaving the pure gold of the child's soul. While none of us would desire for our children to be ill, in our efforts to eradicate all illness with any means necessary we have become materialistic about health and forgotten to see into the subtler nature of our physical experiences.

For all the potential benefit a fever brings, it must be remembered that fevers do signal stress or infection and must be respected. When I was a child my grandma and great-grandma would admonish us to stay home one day extra for each day we had a fever. Of course, I thought this was a hopelessly overprotective tactic to keep me from having fun, but I can now see their wisdom. Too often we send children to school while they are ill or give them very little time at home to recover from illness.

When you do keep your child at home during a fever, you allow him to direct his full energy toward wellness. You avoid more complicated sickness and relapses resulting from incomplete recuperation. You also have the opportunity to nourish him as you look for the cause of the fever. Perhaps all he needs is a break from the stimulation of external activities such as school. In this case, no other symptoms may ever develop, and he will feel better quickly. If other symptoms do develop, you will be on hand to notice them and respond appropriately.

Keeping children at home will naturally present some problems for women with outside jobs. Older children who are not extremely ill can be left at home with emergency phone numbers and perhaps a stay-at-home neighbor to check in on your child. Younger children can perhaps be left under the care of a close friend or relative when your work schedule is inflexible.

THE COURSE OF FEVER

Children's fevers tend to run much higher than those of adults. The height of the temperature does not necessarily reflect the severity of the illness, however. In fact, a child can have a severe disease such as meningitis but only develop a moderate temperature of 101 degrees Fahrenheit. When your child has a fever, providing fluids and rest and attending to any possible infections is more important than being concerned about the degree of the temperature. Fevers may continue for a number of days, as is common with upper respiratory infections and flu, but this is usually not a problem if the child is taking plenty of fluids and resting, the infection is being addressed, and the child's vitality seems strong.

Because fever is the immune system's natural response to stress or infection, when we give fever suppressants, we are confusing the body's instincts. If done repeatedly, long-term consequences may arise. If you are uncomfortable about how hot your child seems and you want to cool him down a bit, place him in a tub of water about two to three degrees cooler than his current body temperature. The child should find the bath comfortable and should not protest that the water is too hot. Anything cooler will be a shock to the system and will defeat your intentions. Alternatively, you could simply apply a cool cloth to the forehead, temples, wrists, and back of the neck.

FEBRILE SEIZURES

Febrile seizures are of great concern to many parents and certainly are incredibly frightening, especially the first time your child goes through one. You may not yet even be aware that your child is feverish when a seizure occurs. Febrile seizures are caused by a rapid change in body temperature, such as when a fever suddenly rises or goes down. The child begins to lose consciousness; spastically moves his arms and legs; and possibly has a bowel movement, urinates, or vomits; the eyes may roll up into the head. Physicians propose that febrile seizures are not dangerous as long as a fever is the cause rather than epilepsy or another neurological problem, and providing breathing is not interrupted during the convulsion. They can be associated with encephalitis or meningitis, so consult your physician should one occur.

During a seizure, turn your child on his side to keep him from choking if he vomits. Be sure that nothing nearby can injure him if he bangs into it. Touch and talk to him to calm and reassure both of you. Loosen any constrictive clothing. The seizure may last up to five minutes, during which time he may shake, roll the eyes and tongue, or convulse. Breathing problems are rare during seizures, but you should make certain that your child is breathing.

A course in CPR may increase your confidence if you have a child prone to febrile seizures. Any seizure that lasts ten minutes or more or one in which breathing stops can cause damage and needs to be brought to the immediate attention of a physician. Febrile seizures, however, rarely pose such a risk, though it is still prudent to have your child seen by your physician.

Closely observe your child after the seizure. Children commonly are quite exhausted and need to sleep. It is fine to let the child sleep, but try to rouse him every fifteen minutes for a few hours to make sure he is conscious and responsive. If it is his first seizure, testing to rule out neurological problems is prudent if you suspect that they may exist.

Febrile seizures tend to recur with subsequent fevers, so you will need to watch the child closely when fevers arise. However, a seizure can be a one-time occurrence. Some doctors recommend medication to control febrile seizures in children who are prone to them, but it is often unnecessary and is potentially harmful to your child. Seek further opinions, and, above all, trust your ability to evaluate the information and decide whether medication seems necessary.

Calm Child Formula (see "Car Sickness") used on a regular basis may prevent seizures because it calms and strengthens the nervous system. Consultation with a practitioner of traditional Chinese medicine may also be helpful, as this age-old system of healing has an excellent reputation for successfully treating chronic problems.

GENERAL RECOMMENDATIONS

- Let your child rest and sleep as much as she needs to. Create a quiet environment conducive to healing and recovery.
- During this time of rest and quiet, provide spirit-lifting activities—for example, read aloud age-appropriate stories if the child is too young to read or doesn't feel up to reading to himself. (*The Secret Garden*, by Frances Hodgson Burnett, is a real winner for reading to kids five years and up.) The television is best left off if possible. It's too stimulating and certainly not as nourishing a companion as you are.
- Keep the child's room fresh and comfortable. Perhaps put a pretty blanket and sheets on the bed and a few plants in the room. Diffuse light, as through a thin curtain on the window, is soothing to feverish eyes.
- To freshen the air, spray the room with a combination of water and a few drops of essential oil in a clean plant mister. Rosemary, lavender, thyme, rose, lemon, eucalyptus, and mint make refreshing scents.

DIETARY RECOMMENDATIONS

- Give your child *loads of fluids* during the fever to prevent dehydration, keep the temperature fairly stable, flush the infection, and ease your child's nerves. Babies can be nursed often and given water by teaspoon, cup, or eyedropper every fifteen to thirty minutes. Older children can drink one cup of liquid every hour, preferably a quarter cup or so every fifteen to thirty minutes. If the child is sleeping, you can rouse him periodically for a drink. Offer a straw to sip through so the child doesn't have to sit up. Herbal teas and dilute juices are fine.
- Keep food light. Fruit, vegetables, soups, and liquids can be given until the fever has broken. Heavy foods contribute heat to the body. However, if a child is hungry, trust his appetite. Stay completely away from cold foods (like ice cream) that may seem comforting but actually exacerbate the problem.

NATURAL THERAPIES DURING FEVERS

- Homeopathic aconite 30x or belladonna 30x are recommended for fevers that have a sudden onset, particularly after the child has been exposed to wind. These can be repeated a few times, about thirty minutes apart, after which some improvement should be noticeable if these particular homeopathic remedies are going to be effective for your child. (Homeopathy is very specific to the individual, and therefore a different remedy may be appropriate. I encourage you to get a copy of *Everybody's Guide to Homeopathic Medicines*, by Stephen Cummings and D. Ullman; see "Further Reading").

- Constipation causes heat to be trapped in the body. If your child seems very hot and dry and has not been having regular bowel movements, refer to "Constipation" earlier in this chapter and begin the appropriate regimens.

  In addition, if the fever is extreme, you may want to try a lukewarm gentle enema of catnip tea. If the fever is high and your child hasn't been drinking much, occasionally, the fluid from the enema will be completely retained. This is fine and can actually be done deliberately to prevent dehydration. NEVER USE COLD WATER IN AN ENEMA—IT CAN LEAD TO SHOCK.

- For achiness, headaches, or restlessness, strong teas of catnip, chamomile, or lemon balm can be used alone or in combination. These herbs are fully safe and gentle, even in large quantities. Baths with these herbs are also soothing. Kudzu-apple juice (see "Colds and Flu") also helps relieve general discomforts. You can also add 5 drops of rosemary oil to a warm bath to bring a sense of restfulness and relieve the above symptoms.

- Catnip, chamomile, and lemon balm soothe tummy upsets, making them ideal for use during fever. Anise seed tea or a weak tea made from fresh gingerroot can quiet indigestion.

- A child who has a fever associated with an infection requires antimicrobial herbs. The following are highly reliable, particularly when used in combination:

  Give echinacea root tincture, 1 drop per 2 pounds of body weight every two to four hours depending on the severity of the illness. Gradually decrease the amount and frequency when the fever subsides, but continue for three more days after the temperature is back to normal. I always give echinacea to my kids when they are feverish because it is a reputable immune-system enhancer.

  Garlic is a supreme ally in all infections and may be used alone or with echinacea as just described. Older children can swallow a clove of finely chopped garlic in a spoonful of honey every four hours. Little children can drink garlic lemonade (see "Chills").

Chickweed, chrysanthemum flowers, and honeysuckle flowers can all be made into infusions that clear heat and reduce infections. Use in conjunction with the above remedies.

- Give vitamin C in addition to herbs to provide extra support in overcoming the illness. Give 250 to 500 milligrams every four hours, depending upon the age of the child and the severity of the illness. Vitamin C is not toxic, but large doses will cause loose stools. Kale, alfalfa sprouts, rosehips, and violet leaves and blossoms are also rich in vitamin C and can be added to the diet. If you want to give your child orange juice, give only juice that is fresh-squeezed at home and kept at room temperature. Oranges have a tendency to aggravate stomach upsets and increase mucus production. They are also a tropical, cold-natured fruit that is best avoided during fevers, especially during cold weather.

REDUCING FEVERS

Most often fevers will abate on their own, so all you need to do is support the child and treat the underlying causes. There are times, though, when we become anxious at how high the fever is or how long it is going on. Or perhaps your child seems so uncomfortable that you want to give some temporary relief. Herbs offer an effective means of reducing fevers without side effects. Many of the herbs that are useful for common discomforts with fever also reduce fever.

- *Peppermint leaf and elder blossom infusion:* Steep 1/2 ounce of each herb in a covered quart jar of boiling water for twenty minutes. Strain and sweeten if necessary. Give as warm as the child will take it, and often, until a sweat results.
- *Catnip infusion:* Prepare as above with 1 ounce of catnip to 1 quart of water.
- *Lemon balm infusion:* Use 2 ounces of herb to 1 quart of water, as above. This is very pleasant tasting and very gentle, even for little babies.

Note that mothers of feverish nursing babies should themselves take adult dosages of these remedies. Some of the benefits of the herbs will pass through your milk to the baby.

MENINGITIS AND FEVER

Parents often fearfully equate meningitis with fever, particularly high fever. However, most fevers are not caused by meningitis, and when meningitis does strike, the child may not have a high fever at all; it may be only in the range of 101–102 degrees Fahrenheit. Therefore, the best thing you can do is to be aware of the general symptoms of this illness in addition to fever. Though it is not a common illness, it is important to be aware of it because bacterial meningitis can be seriously and permanently disabling, and many times it is fatal. See also "Meningitis."

WHEN TO SEEK MEDICAL CARE

If you are concerned about or suspect meningitis, seek medical help immediately. Antibiotics and medical treatment are definitely warranted here. Signs of meningitis include fever (or sometimes a subnormal temperature), stiffness or soreness of the neck (test to see if the child experiences discomfort when trying to press his chin to his chest), listlessness, vomiting, poor eating, inconsolable crying or irritability in very young children, headache, or resistance to being held. There may be an unusual rash. Newborns may not have any specific symptoms but seem generally ill. One sign in babies is a bulging fontanel, the soft spot on top of the head. Older children may have many symptoms or just a few.)

❖ GERMAN MEASLES (RUBELLA) ❖

German measles is a viral infection common in childhood. The symptoms are similar to measles but can be so mild that the illness is barely noticeable. The rash may be a little itchy. The incubation period is two to three weeks, and it is considered highly contagious. While rubella poses no threat to children, it is a great problem for unborn babies. If a pregnant woman becomes infected with this virus, particularly during the first trimester, miscarriage or severe congenital deformities may result. To prevent it, girls can be exposed to the illness or given the rubella vaccination prior to child-bearing age. This will usually provide enough protection, but a simple blood test can verify whether immunity has been conferred. If an adult woman chooses to be vaccinated for German measles, she should wait three months before becoming pregnant. This vaccine sometimes causes temporary arthritis in adult women. Any children known to be exposed to German measles should be kept at home until the illness has passed and should avoid contact with pregnant women during this time.

Treatment of German measles, if it is necessary, should be based upon the remedies for measles.

❖ Headaches ❖

Young children usually do not have more than an occasional headache, but older children and teenagers are likely to develop them more frequently in response to emotional stress, increasing pressures at home or school, and the physical and emotional changes of puberty. The years prior to and during puberty are sensitive times, requiring parents to find a balance between involvement in their children's lives and giving them space and privacy. If your child is having mild headaches, talk to him or her to help with stress reduction and diet (inadequate nutrition and junk foods as well as constipation can contribute to headaches), and listen to anything he or she may want to share with you.

Eyestrain is sometimes a cause of headaches. Provide your child with good light for reading, homework, and other projects, and learn about exercises for strengthening eyes. Encourage your child to go to sleep at a reasonable hour. If necessary, consult an eye doctor.

Severe headaches that recur often; headaches associated with a head injury; or severe headache accompanied by fever, vomiting, or stiff neck can indicate serious conditions requiring prompt medical care.

General Recommendations

- Minerals keep the nervous system strong. If your child is getting headaches, see if she is eating mineral-rich foods on a regular basis. Yogurt, vegetables, nuts, seeds, and seaweeds all provide minerals. Add these foods to the diet along with infusions of nettles as a daily supplement. Kelp powder, up to 1 tablespoon daily in food or in capsules, can also supply essential dietary elements.
- Massage is often overlooked as a therapeutic modality but is in fact effective, safe, and comforting. Headaches are especially responsive to simple massage techniques. Don't let a lack of professional training discourage you from rubbing your child's neck, shoulders, and head. Done twice a week, it can prevent headaches and is a wonderful way to help your child when a headache does occur. Teach your child to do self-massage by having her rub the area over the bridge of the nose, the eyebrows, and the temples at the onset of a headache.
- Like massage, visualization is an effective and gentle technique. There are a number of books on this subject, even some specifically geared toward children, which can teach you how to use this technique during illnesses or for discomforts. Refer to "Further Reading" for titles.

- Chamomile is a gentle analgesic, perfect for headaches and general relaxation at any age. It is also rich in calcium and minerals that nourish the nervous system. To drink as a tea, steep 1 tablespoon of herb in 1 cup hot water for twenty minutes. Strain and sweeten if desired. Use as needed. The lovely scent of an herbal pillow made with chamomile can help a child with a headache drift into a peaceful sleep (see "Nightmares and Sleep Disturbances").
- Other herbs noted for their effectiveness in treating headaches are catnip, lemon balm, rosemary, skullcap, vervain, valerian, and lavender. These can be used alone or in combination as teas or tinctures. To use the tinctures as a tonic, give approximately 15 drops in water twice a day; during an acute headache, give 5 to 10 drops every thirty minutes. To use as a drink, prepare standard tea and give up to 2 cups daily.
- Add a few drops of oil of lavender or rosemary to a bath for relaxation.

❖ HEAD INJURIES ❖

The skull is quite strong and the brain well protected, so mild blows to the head usually require no care other than comforting and watching your child. Large bumps can be rubbed with arnica oil if the skin is unbroken, calendula oil if there are any abrasions or cuts. Homeopathic arnica 30x can be given immediately to prevent swelling and to minimize bruising or trauma. Bach Rescue Remedy (4 drops, repeated as necessary) calms a hysterical child.

WHEN TO SEEK MEDICAL CARE

SEVERE BLOWS OR ACCIDENTS THAT LEAD TO UNCON-SCIOUSNESS REQUIRE IMMEDIATE EMERGENCY MEDICAL HELP. If you see any of the following signs of cerebral hemorrhage, GET YOUR CHILD TO AN EMERGENCY ROOM IMMEDI-ATELY: stiff neck, worsening headache, unequal dilation of the pupils, repeated vomiting, change in consciousness, abdominal pain, vision problems, numbness of any parts of the body, seizures, or bleeding from the ears. These signs will usually occur within twenty-four hours of the injury but can appear for up to two weeks after.

Children often feel tired after an accident and want to sleep. This is normal and fine, but you should try to wake the child about every fifteen minutes for the first hour and periodically thereafter to be certain that he is conscious and not displaying any danger signs.

Even small cuts on the scalp can bleed profusely, often making the injury appear worse than it is. Rinse the area thoroughly to evaluate the extent of the cut, and apply pressure to minimize the bleeding. Seek help if the injury is extensive, if the bleeding is uncontrollable or severe, or if the injury was caused by an unclean object and you think your child requires a tetanus shot.

❖ HYPERACTIVITY ❖

Children are naturally inclined to be energetic, physically active, and free spirited. Situations that require them to be still and concentrate for long periods of time go against these tendencies. Staying indoors for so much of the day, as they are when in school, is especially unnatural for them. Viewed in this way, hyperactivity is not something wrong with children. It is sometimes a lifestyle problem and frequently a "social problem." Ironically, hyperactivity is a modern phenomenon that occurs mostly among school-age children, and frequently it is first "diagnosed" by teachers.

Even more ironic, children labeled as hyperactive or with learning disorders are often required to take their medication *only* on school days. On this basis alone, we must surely begin to question whether the medication is for the intrinsic benefit of the student or if our educational system is failing to provide learning opportunities that meet the unique and diverse needs of our children. We've created packaged education, "McLearning," as one educator has put it, and the kids who don't fit into the Happy Meal box don't get served—they get rejected from the assembly line as unpackageable products. If they don't fit, they must be made to. Medications create compliance and docility in these children and give the superficial appearance that the children are fitting, but really, they are being cheated.

Hyperactivity and attention-deficit disorder are real disorders, of course, but we need to be cautious about their identification. Today, the terms are overused and popularized to the point where they are thrown about too easily and children may be categorized erroneously.

If medications are being recommended to modify your child's behavior, evaluate the situation. Ask yourself if the expectations being placed on him are appropriate for his age, needs, and personality. Some children may learn more effectively in less-traditional settings where they can move around or work at their own pace. If possible, look into educational programs that are supportive of your child's individual needs before you allow him to be labeled and medicated.

Schools like the Waldorf Schools incorporate movement, individualized attention, and time outdoors into the daily schedule. Homeschooling is also becoming a more commonly accepted option that allows your child the greatest individualized attention and the space to be himself and to learn in a nonpressured way. For more information, refer to "Further Reading."

If your child's school is the only option, see if your child's teacher is willing to incorporate periodic breaks for physical activity into the schoolday. Encourage your child to play outside after school, and give encouragement and assistance with schoolwork if your child is having academic difficulty. Remember that every child has a unique way of learning and learns at his or her own pace.

Dietary additives and environmental pollutants (including food colorings, preservatives, pesticide residues, caffeine, sugar, and heavy metals) can irritate your child's nerves and adrenal glands, resulting in the irritability, boundless movement, lack of focus on tasks, and aggressive behavior characteristic of hyperactivity. Eliminate as many of these substances as possible from your child's surroundings and foods. *Non-Toxic and Natural*, by Deborah Lynn Dodd, can provide you with information on preparing and obtaining natural household products and cleaners. In "Further Reading" you can also find books about natural foods and healthy eating. Replacing synthetic and processed foods with high-quality nourishment for your family really is not too difficult. *Superimmunity for Kids*, by Leo Galland, will give you insights into the connection between a child's diet and behavior.

Children are great imitators; they internalize what they see and reflect it back. Stresses at home and even images on television can contribute to unsettled, aggressive behavior. The vivid images of television programs combined with inactivity while watching them leads to bottled-up energy that children may later release chaotically. Cut back on TV or get rid of it altogether. You'll find that when it is not a regular part of life, you'll get to know your family better!

Children who are having trouble relaxing or concentrating can benefit from a discipline such as yoga, tai chi or other martial arts, as well as from learning the art of creative visualization or meditation. See "Further Reading" for titles of books on these subjects.

Counseling may be helpful if the relationships or problems at home are longstanding and seem to be affecting your child's well-being.

HERBAL RECOMMENDATIONS

Herbs that support and nourish the nerves and glandular system are particularly appropriate here. Also helpful are herbs that are rich in nutrients and those that help eliminate heavy metals and other environmental toxins. Most of these produce mild relaxation—they do not act as sedatives or narcotics. Occasionally you can give stronger, more sedating doses to help a child rest or sleep (see "Nightmares and Sleep Disturbances"). Unless otherwise noted, you can use these herbs regularly over a long period of time as tonics. Choose a couple of nervines to use in combination with the nutritive and blood-purifying herbs. Remember that change takes time, and that herbal therapies must be accompanied by lifestyle changes.

NERVINES

- Oats are rich in calcium, strengthen the nervous system, and are mildly sedating. Most children enjoy oatmeal, muesli, oatcakes, and other foods prepared with oats. Infusions of oatstraw are also beneficial and pleasant tasting. Steep 1 heaping tablespoon per cup of boiling water for thirty minutes, flavoring it with fennel, anise, orange peel, lemon grass, licorice, or any other herb your child likes. The "flavoring" herbs just mentioned have the additional benefit of aiding digestion, which also quiets the nerves. In Ayurvedic medicine, excess "vata," or "wind," aggravates the nerves, thereby creating hyperexcitability. These herbs are considered wind-eliminating herbs. Oats are specifically used for pacifying the vata.
- Catnip, chamomile, and lemon balm are the herbs of choice for children with irritability and hyperactivity. Daily cupfuls of tea can become a familiar and pleasant ritual for you and your children to share and can replace juice and other sugary beverages in the diet.
- Calm Child Formula, in infusion and tincture form, is slightly stronger than these teas but is still safe and gentle as a nutritive tonic used daily and over a long time. A wonderful nervine and digestive calmer, it helps bring the child a sense of tranquility. It can be purchased in a tincture form under the "Planetary Formulas" label or can be prepared at home as an infusion or syrup (see "Car Sickness").
- Skullcap, valerian, and hops are relaxing herbs that can provide both immediate and long-term benefits. Use individually or in combination in small, regular doses of 5 to 15 drops of tincture daily.

- Motherwort is a very bitter but soothing herb that can be given occasionally. Use 3 to 10 drops of the tincture in water or in a quarter teaspoon of honey. Daily use is discouraged, so do not use it more than a few times a week.

BLOOD PURIFYING AND NUTRITIVE HERBS

These are used to eliminate heavy metals and other environmental contaminants from the body and to provide high-quality minerals.

- Red clover is a common garden weed regarded for its ability to "cleanse" the blood. It supplies trace minerals and is also mildly antispasmodic, meaning that it eases nervous excitability, twitching, and spasm. Prepare as an infusion, 1 ounce per pint of boiling water. Steep for one hour. Dosage is 1 cup daily, hot or cold, by itself or mixed with other herbs.

- Kelp is an incredibly strong and flexible sea plant. Chemical components in kelp enable it to bind heavy metals and radioactive substances and to quickly eliminate them from the body through the bowels. In Europe, kelp is reportedly used by workers at nuclear power plants as a preventive measure against radiation poisoning. In addition, kelp helps regulate the glandular system. It is an excellent source of iodine and is also rich in vitamins B, D, E, and K and the minerals calcium and magnesium. It is very useful for nervous disorders in children and adults alike.

    Kelp may be used in all the following ways and on a regular basis: sprinkle the powder, up to 1 tablespoon daily, on foods; give up to 6 "00" capsules filled with the powder daily; cook pieces of whole kelp (Kombu) in beans, soups, and stews; make kelp tea by boiling a 6- to 8-inch strip of kelp in 2 cups water for thirty minutes. Drink the broth plain or flavored with bouillon or miso paste.

    A taste for kelp may need to be acquired over time, so start with very small amounts. But stick with it because it is so very beneficial.

- Nettles stabilizes blood sugar, strengthens adrenal function, and reduces allergy problems, among other things. A plant chock full of minerals and vitality, it energizes the user but the type of energy one derives from it is steady and stable. One cup daily of infusion will enhance your child's general well-being and balance erratic blood sugar, which could be leading to emotional irritability and behavioral difficulty. In the spring, you can cook young nettles and serve them as a vegetable.

- Another "cool-out" herb for aggressive outbursts is dandelion root. This is an excellent liver tonic, a digestive aid, and a boon to healthy elimination. In addition, dandelion provides trace nutrients from the soil. The infusion is too strong tasting for most kids, so make a syrup and give 1 tablespoon a day, or use 10 to 30 drops of tincture twice a day. Continue for a minimum of six weeks, watching for improvement during this time. Dandelion is safe to give on a regular, ongoing basis; so if improvements are noticeable, you may want to use this herb as a regular dietary supplement.

❖ Impetigo ❖

Patches or spots of infected sores are often a symptom of impetigo. The sores develop as small, fluid-filled spots and then change into pus-filled, runny, or crusty lesions. They most commonly appear on the legs and arms but may be seen on other areas of the body. Impetigo most frequently occurs in hot, humid climates and is usually the consequence of kids scratching mosquito bites or picking at scabs with dirty hands. *Staphylococcus* or *Streptococcus* organisms are generally associated with the infection, which is highly contagious.

Good hygiene will both prevent infection and prevent the spread of infection should it occur. Children can be taught to not pick at their sores and to wash hands regularly. Let them know that this will not only help them but also help prevent infection of other people.

The skin is a large part of the body's immune system, keeping a healthy balance between our internal environment and the organisms that naturally surround us. Skin infections may indicate that the body's defense mechanisms need strengthening. An immediate approach to impetigo is to reduce the external infection and the discomforts that accompany it. Beyond this, you need to build the child's immunity and teach basic hygiene. The recommendations below focus on relief of the immediate condition. Use a combination of internal and external remedies.

Internal Remedies for Impetigo

- Alteratives, herbs that assist the immune system, cool the blood, and are antimicrobial, will be needed. Excellent choices here include echinacea, plantain, burdock root, astragalus, chickweed, propolis, and garlic. Nasturtium leaves and flowers are said to be excellent in the treatment of staph infections. All these herbs are quite safe and can be used alone or in combination, in infusion or tincture. Dosage is 15 to 30 drops of tincture four times a day or 2 to 4 cups of infusion daily.

- Depending upon the child's age, give 150 to 500 milligrams of vitamin C four times a day in addition to the herbs.
- As with all infections, the child should drink plenty of water.
- The diet should consist of fresh vegetables, whole grains, easy-to-digest proteins, and fruit. Reduce the consumption of dairy foods, fatty or red meat, and peanut butter until the infection has cleared. Carrot, beet, and other fresh vegetable juices (to which fresh juiced apples can be added for flavor) are especially good in the treatment of impetigo.

External Remedies for Impetigo

- Wash the sores a few times a day with a rinse of calendula infusion or dilute calendula tincture. To dilute the tincture, mix 1 tablespoon in 1 cup water.
- Other herbs that may be added to a wash include myrrh, lavender, echinacea, goldenseal, chickweed, burdock root, rosemary, plantain, and thyme.
- After washing, sprinkle powdered slippery elm, chaparral, myrrh, or goldenseal, alone or in combination, on oozing sores to absorb the pus, promoting their drying and healing.
- For sores that form a crust or are especially itchy, salve containing calendula provides healing and comfort. Substitute calendula oil if you don't have salve.
- The use of salve or oil also prevents scarring.

❖ Infections (General) ❖

Excellent nutrition, plenty of rest, fresh air, exercise, and healthy elimination keep children strong and enable them to deal with occasional illnesses without harm. This section discusses ways to prevent infection. Because an infection can affect the body in so many ways, this book discusses particular conditions in other sections; refer to the table of contents.

When children are under stress, traveling, or teething, or if they have been exposed to someone who is ill, they can be given herbs to prevent illness. Echinacea is an excellent choice as a preventive measure. Give 10 to 20 drops of the tincture a couple of times a day. Garlic, also a preventive remedy, can be given in the form of perles (soft pills filled with concentrated garlic oil), syrup, or garlic lemonade (see "Chills"), or in its raw, fresh state, finely chopped and added to a teaspoon of honey.

Often, children who are prone to infection and frequent illness need to have their diets changed or bolstered to include foods that are more nutritious and more in harmony with the seasons and the needs of their particular bodies. Lack of essential nutrients leaves the body unable to motivate itself to a state of optimal health and resistance to illness. Likewise, eating unhealthy foods diminishes the body's optimal functioning capacity. Use your intuition, read about diet and nutrition, and provide a wide variety of nutritious foods from which your family can choose.

A balance between ample physical activity and adequate rest is so important that it cannot be overstated. Children desire a lot of activity and movement. These are essential for good digestion, circulation, metabolism, and oxygenation of the body, all of the factors that enable children to make use of nutrients and thrive. Of course, fun is also an ingredient in this recipe.

Physical activity aids sleep, too, though many children once past the age of about three or four years old will begin to resist sleep, even when tired. It is up to you to help them learn to identify the need for rest and quiet times. When a child is perpetually exhausted, he or she is most likely to become ill. When we are overstimulated, our psychic forces are so busy processing our experiences that our resistance to illness is reduced. By providing times for outward worldly activity, adequate sleep, and inward, calm, reflective time, even just for a short time each day, you will teach your child to respect the rhythms of her body. This is a gift that will teach your child to respect her inner needs even as worldly demands increase.

Regular massage as well as the use of moxabustion (as described in "Bed-Wetting") can also mobilize vitality and improve your child's resistance to illness.

WHEN TO SEEK MEDICAL CARE

Obtain immediate medical care for any of the following conditions: External infections that resist improvement or that are accompanied by foul odor, red streaks, fever, or general systemic illness. Internal infections with fever accompanied by stiff neck and/or projectile vomiting; persistent fever with no overall improvement; abnormally low temperature, especially when accompanied by listlessness; sharp abdominal pain; bulging soft spot in a newborn or baby; breathing difficulty; extreme and persistent diarrhea or vomiting; loss of consciousness.

❖ INTESTINAL PARASITES ❖

While it may be an unpleasant aspect of our humanity, as members of an ecosystem that includes a variety of creatures large and small, visible and invisible, we are host at any given time to innumerable organisms. Intestinal parasites can at times be among them.

In most temperate climates, intestinal worms are generally not life threatening to hosts with adequate diet and hygiene. The worms most likely to be picked up in the United States include pinworms (also called "threadworms" or "seatworms"), roundworms, hookworms, and tapeworms. Fortunately, the last three are fairly rare. Following you will find general descriptions of parasitic infestations as well as guidelines for preventing infection and a general section on treatments.

Tapeworms are picked up by eating undercooked, contaminated meats and fish. These worms attach themselves to the lining of the intestines and over time can pose a serious health threat. Initial symptoms of tapeworm infection are stomach aches. Occasionally flat, white pieces of the worm, less than an inch in length, can be seen in the stools. Prevention calls for thorough cooking of all meat and fish and care in the cleaning of kitchen utensils used in their preparation.

Hookworms are about a centimeter long and are red in color. They infect a person when the baby worms, which live in the soil, enter through a person's bare feet. Hookworms occur mainly in the southeastern United States and in the tropics. Symptoms include itchy feet initially, then diarrhea, stomach ache, dry coughing, weakness, eating of dirt, and anemia. The eggs are eliminated through the stools, which can then reinfect the soil. Infection can be determined through an analysis of a stool sample (the local health department usually offers this service). These worms can severely weaken a child. Prevention includes wearing shoes, particularly in areas that have been sites for human and animal wastes, as well as careful sanitation and hygiene.

Roundworms can grow to be quite large, up to 10 inches or more. They are usually seen only after travels to semitropical and tropical areas (for example, the Caribbean or Mexico), where they are picked up by eating contaminated foods. Usually, the only symptoms are a dry cough, generalized itching, and a bellyache. The abdomen may appear swollen. The child may become weak as the worms multiply and sap the energy. In severe cases, they can cause pneumonia, intestinal obstruction, or airway blockage if they travel in the body. Prevention includes excellent hygiene, protection of food from flies, care in eating when traveling, and promotion of strong digestion and elimination.

Pinworms are white worms about 1 centimeter long that look like tiny threads. They can cause some or all of the following symptoms: anal itching, vaginal itching or pain, night waking, irritability at bedtime or even during the day, constipation, chronic dry cough, nose picking, dark circles under the eyes, strong appetite for sweets, whininess, and belly-aches that may be mild or intense. These symptoms may come and go in cycles every few weeks to months. While pinworms are not dangerous, they are very common among school-age children, highly transmittable, and draining to the vitality of children. They are nearly ubiquitous: Statistics indicate that anywhere from 10 to 90 percent of the American population may carry them. They are a common problem among affluent middle-class families, primarily with young children. The worms are spread by eggs that are picked up in a variety of ways: from the fingers of kids or adults who have scratched their bottoms and not washed their hands; from contaminated clothing and linens; from contaminated food; from the soil or the sandbox. The eggs, which can remain dormant for months, are even said to be airborne. Detection can be through a stool sample, or, more simply, you can look at your child's anus with a flashlight after he or she has gone to sleep—often the worms are visible. Prevention lies primarily in hygiene and catching the problem early, along with attention to diet and digestive health.

REMEDIES FOR INTESTINAL PARASITES

Herbs and medications that destroy and eliminate worms are called "anthelmintics" and "vermifuges." Herbs used for this purpose tend to be painfully bitter or spicy—too much so for young children. In addition, they must be taken in sufficiently large quantities to be effective. Medical treatment for worms involves the use of strong chemicals, some derived from plants and some synthetic, but usually they need to be taken in at most a few concentrated doses. In some cases only one dose is required. Since tapeworms, hookworms, and even roundworms can cause significant health problems and are very hard to eliminate (you could not safely get your child to consume anywhere near enough of the necessary herbs to address the problem), a pharmaceutical drug is the treatment of choice. Although the medications are also poisons, they come in carefully measured amounts, and following the instructions should give you good results with no harm. Natural home remedies can occasionally eliminate roundworms. You may want to do this by following the pinworm regime for a chosen time, then reevaluate the need for drugs. Do not use worm treatment herbs and medications at the same time.

REMEDIES FOR PINWORMS

Pinworms can be very challenging to eliminate with herbal remedies, but with persistence and scrupulous attention to hygiene, it can be done. The worms have a life cycle of approximately two weeks, so the real trick to eliminating them is preventing reinfestation. If you are able to do this, you can clear up the problem in three to six weeks. If the problem persists after a number of attempts with natural remedies, a standard medication (such as Vermox) may be the best solution because a pinworm infestation can be very bothersome to a young child. In fact, even the medication *without the hygienic measures* often fail to prevent reinfestation, so no matter what you choose to do observe the following guidelines. Note that when one member of a family is infected, it is likely that all members have or will shortly have them and should be treated also. This is important to keep in mind because Vermox and other medications are not safe for pregnant women and children under two years.

GENERAL CARE AND HYGIENE

- First and foremost, it is essential that your family join together in the effort to prevent reinfestation. If the family works as a team, it will be far less of a demanding chore. Try to enlist everyone's goodwill and assistance. While hygiene and housekeeping are crucial, the family should not internalize the problem as "we're dirty." That is not the point at all, and that thought process undermines your family's ability to deal with the tasks at hand.
- Remember, if one person in the family is infected, treat everyone to prevent successive infections.
- Thoroughly wash hands before preparing food, and get children into the habit of washing hands with warm, soapy water upon awakening and before all meals.
- Keeping fingernails short will prevent the eggs from having a place to collect if you have any bottom scratchers or nose pickers in the family. This practice is very important in preventing reinfection. Teach family members that if they do scratch, they should wash hands and under nails immediately, and remind them to stop scratching!
- Get kids (and adults) to wear underwear or close-fitting bottoms to bed. This will prevent eggs and critters from getting very far.
- Change bath towels after each use, and launder hand towels every couple of days.
- Change all bedding every three days. Don't shake out the sheets as you take them off the bed as this will send the tiny eggs flying. Just fold up the sheets and wash on a hot cycle.

- Vacuum (DON'T sweep) every couple of days, and damp-mop at least once a week. Clean around the toilet and wipe faucets and doorknobs in the bathroom every couple of days.

This is a hefty regime, but if you want to avoid using medication, it is your best bet.

GENERAL RECOMMENDATIONS

- This first remedy is probably the single most effective solution I know of, and it is (yay!) simple. It also brings relief to an itching bottom. Every night (either before your child goes to sleep or after if doing this will embarrass the child) paint a glob of petroleum jelly (Vaseline) onto and around your child's anus (a diameter of about a half-dollar will do). Some suggest zinc oxide (available in the pharmacy) instead, but it absorbs too easily; petroleum jelly is more effective. You must do this every night during the active phase of the outbreak and, ideally, every night for a total of four to six weeks. This is an excellent way to keep the female from laying eggs, thereby breaking the cycle of infection. You must repeat the remedy for the full time period to prevent the eggs from maturing and then the new females from laying.

- To treat vaginal pinworms (your daughter will complain of itching or pain or will scratch at her bottom during the day or as she is going to sleep), apply salve or petroleum jelly to the area of her labia and her perineum (the fleshy area between the vaginal opening and the anus) to reduce discomfort (she can do this herself if modesty is a concern) and repeat the application at night. Every day, give her a bath to which you add 1 cup of Epsom salts. She should find relief within three days.

- Teach girls to wipe from front to back after using the toilet to prevent spreading the eggs (and other germs as well). Be sure to address the possibility of urinary-tract infection, which may crop up with vaginal pinworms. Symptoms include frequent or painful urination, sometimes accompanied by chills, nausea, or soreness of the lower abdomen or lower back.

DIETARY RECOMMENDATIONS

- Hygiene in the kitchen is the most beneficial remedy. Wash before meals; clean all fresh fruits and vegetables well, especially those that grow in or close to the soil; and get kids to use utensils instead of fingers for eating. Sharing food with other kids should be avoided so that your family isn't passing the problem along or picking it back up. Avoid serving finger foods during an outbreak.

- Even with a healthy diet, pinworms happen. However, deemphasizing certain foods and emphasizing others can help eliminate them or prevent their recurrence.

  Decrease or eliminate refined foods such as white flour and other highly processed products, baked goods, sweets (including natural ones), juices, and even the amount of fruit in the diet.

  Increase or emphasize high-quality, nondairy protein; whole grains; and fresh vegetables, particularly those high in calcium and vitamin A such as leafy greens (kale, collards, mustard greens, broccoli), carrots (and carrot juice), squashes, and sea vegetables (dulse, kelp, hijiki). Calcium and vitamin A apparently help increase resistance to intestinal parasites.
- Certain foods are considered irritating and discouraging to worms. These include pickles, apple cider vinegar, salty foods, onions, garlic, hot peppers, and calamyrna figs. You may want to increase the spiciness of your diet for a while.
- Raw pumpkin seeds are considered a pinworm remedy par excellence. Let kids munch handfuls here and there, and add them to salad, oatmeal, and other foods. Up to a cup a day for school-age children is ideal, but less is, of course, better than none.
- Vegetarian kids may possibly be more susceptible to pinworms owing to what colleagues and I have speculated is a low level of hydrochloric acid in the stomach. Stomach HCl destroys the eggs, and vegetarians may have lower levels of this acid in the stomach. If your family is strictly vegetarian and you are having chronic problems with pinworms, you may want to think about adding small amounts of meat to your diet or speak with a nutritionist about ways you can raise the HCl levels.
- Digestive weakness in anyone can predispose them to parasites. Most kids will outgrow susceptibility to pinworms by age seven, perhaps because they naturally begin to observe better hygiene, spend less time playing in the soil and sand, and stop putting things into their mouths. Major Six Herbs Combination, a Chinese herbal formula for strengthening "digestive fire" in children, may help. It is available through Brion Herbs (see "Resources").

HERBAL RECOMMENDATIONS

The following herbal medicaments are variably effective but may be included in a combination of your choice as part of an overall approach. Some are painfully bitter and are listed in case you want to try them with older children, but don't force unpleasant-tasting worming remedies on your kids. While bitter herbs have an important place in the elimination of pinworms, their strong flavor may be nature's way of protecting us from overconsuming these plants, many of which are rich in potentially toxic alkaloids.

- Garlic is a time-honored medicine for killing worms. It can be taken in garlic lemonade (see "Chills"), perles, or it may even be rubbed onto bare feet that have first been wiped with vegetable oil (though this use of garlic has occasionally caused blistering to sensitive feet!), but is most likely to be effective when eaten raw. As much as possible should be given, up to six raw cloves to older children. Obviously, this is a lot and some is better than none. Garlic can be chopped finely or put through a garlic press and swallowed in a spoonful of apple juice or honey, or added to soup, salad, or other dishes. Repeat as often as possible during the active phase of the infestation and every few days during the dormant phase. Keep in mind that too much garlic is going to make a kid's stomach feel lousy!
- Homeopathic cina 30x is often recommended. It is prepared from the plant called "wormseed." Repeat three times a day during active infection, and less often during the dormant phase. Homeopathic remedies work more to strengthen the constitution of the child than to actually eliminate the worms, so they should be an adjunct to another therapeutic method.
- Black walnut tincture, 10 to 20 drops two to three times a day, or false unicorn root tincture, 10 to 15 drops twice daily, may be effective in the elimination of this problem. The latter is quite bitter, but because it is a tincture the concentrated drops can be disguised in a food or beverage. Applesauce is a great medium for bitter tinctures, according to one friend of mine with a toddler.
- Aloe vera is an easy-to-grow houseplant that yields a juice that heals burns. It is also an intestinal purgative taken internally in large amounts. Midwife Sher Willis (Wonshe) shared the following remedy for getting rid of pinworms: Break off a very thin piece of the aloe plant. The length should equal the end section of the child's pinkie finger. Twice a day for seven days, have the child swallow a piece this size whole. After a week, repeat for three days; after another week, repeat for three more days.

  If your child has trouble swallowing it whole, chop it into fine pieces and place them in the end of a drinking straw. As your child sips a drink through the straw, he or she will swallow the aloe.
- Wormwood is a dreadfully bitter and potentially toxic herb that is generally included in worm remedies. It is taken in an infusion

of 1/2 ounce of herb to 1 quart of water. Standard dose is 1 cup daily for five days. Repeat for two days in the next two consecutive weeks. Wormweed is fairly unpalatable to most adults, not to mention kids, and it's nearly impossible to give a sufficient quantity to be effective. A worm medication is preferable.

- Laxative herbs such as fennel seeds and plantain seeds may assist the body in expelling worms. Fennel can be taken as a tea to reduce bellyaches and gas. Plantain seeds, which are similar to flax seeds, can be gathered in the autumn or purchased at an herb shop or health-food store that sells herbs. Take 1 tablespoon daily for a few weeks. They can be sprinkled in foods, eaten raw, or made into a paste by grinding them with honey and nut butter.
- Seeds from the papaya fruit contain enzymes believed to destroy worms as well as aid digestion. Natural-food stores usually sell them in chewable tablets, which are sweet, making this a good remedy to follow a less-palatable one as an incentive for kids. Because papaya seeds work by breaking down animal proteins, it may be best to decrease meat and dairy products during the treatment period. Give according to the dosage recommended for the product you purchase, every day for four to six weeks.

Remember not to guilt-trip yourself or your family if you need to use a prescription drug. Everything has its place. With persistence and carefully observed hygiene, however, you stand a good chance of eliminating this problem naturally.

❖ IRRITABILITY ❖

Irritability, crankiness, and whining are most likely to occur when a child is tired or hungry. It may also be the first obvious sign that your child is becoming sick. Other causes of irritability include overstimulation, consuming too much sugar or fruit juice, deficiency of minerals (especially calcium), and intestinal parasites (particularly pinworms). Parasites further aggravate a mineral deficiency. General nutrition is important to consider as well. Because children are growing so fast, they need a diet rich in high-quality foods that provide them with the nutrients they require. Adequate protein and carbohydrate intake is necessary to keep the blood sugar steady, preventing the mood swings characteristic of hypoglycemia. Herbs can serve as a supplementary part of the diet. Nettles is especially helpful for keeping the blood sugar stable and, as an infusion, it provides many minerals.

When your child is cranky, help him or her relax and sleep, and take lots of time for cuddles. If you suspect a cold coming on, give a bit of echinacea tincture or garlic lemonade (see "Chills") to boost the immune system. Calm Child Formula (see "Car Sickness") and other nervines such as catnip, lemon balm, and skullcap teas are great for helping your child calm down. Hops tincture, 10 to 15 drops, can get your child to sleep if he's wound up and overtired. Massage using an herbal massage oil or a bath with a few drops of essential oil in the tub is also calming and soothing. Rose and lavender oils are nice choices. Laughter, of course, is always a great way to "un-crank" someone!

In addition to the herbs listed above, the following help calm an irritable child: chamomile, slippery elm, lemon grass, marshmallow root, oatstraw, lime blossom, and catnip. Feel free to create your own blends. Optional flavoring additions include rosehips, cinnamon, peppermint, fennel, and licorice root. Herbal baths can be made with any of the calming herbs listed above. The act of drinking a cup of warm tea is, in itself, calming and relaxing, as are herbal baths.

See "Hyperactivity" for other ideas.

❖ Lice ❖

These small mites live on the scalp and survive by drawing their food from our blood. Lice are visible to the naked eye and so are their tiny eggs, called "nits," which they lay at the base of the hair. Lice cause intense itching in most cases, and outbreaks are prevalent among schoolchildren.

During an outbreak, follow the suggestions for preventing infestation. Should an infestation occur, diligent application of the following treatments should successfully eliminate it.

PREVENTION

Lice are highly contagious. They can actually jump from one person to another, so anyone with an infestation should keep a distance from others to prevent its spreading. Personal items such as hats, brushes, and pillows should not be shared. Wearing a hair covering like a bandanna also minimizes the chance of infesting others. When one person in a family has lice, everyone should do at least of couple of washes with herbs. Check scalps so you can stay on top of further outbreaks.

HERBAL RECOMMENDATIONS

- Mix 4 cups apple cider vinegar, 4 cups water, and 1/2 ounce of essential oil of thyme. Massage the mixture into the scalp and rinse the hair with it nightly. Use 1/2 cup for children seven and over, 1/4 cup for younger children. Be *very careful to keep it out of the eyes* as it burns, although it is not dangerous. Also avoid ingestion.

You can replace the thyme oil with the herb. Steep 2 ounces of thyme for an hour in the 4 cups of water (which must be boiling hot); then add with the vinegar. Other oils that can be used in place of thyme oil are sassafras, anise seed, and lavender, although thyme seems particularly effective. Repeat each night for one week.

- After each rinsing, apply some olive or coconut oil to the scalp to prevent dryness and to loosen the nits. Cover the hair with a scarf or bandanna at night, and rinse or shampoo in the morning.
- Comb the hair daily with a fine-toothed comb (available at any pharmacy), picking out as many lice and eggs as possible.
- Thoroughly wash and dry all clothing, towels, and linens every two days, using hot water.
- Repeat the treatment for an additional two days each week for two weeks to kill any eggs that have possibly lingered and hatched.

Common treatment for lice includes the use of either Kwell or pyrethrin-based substances. Kwell contains strong and harmful chemicals. Even one application using too much can lead to serious nervous-system damage and convulsions in a young child. Pyrethrins come from chrysanthemums and are safe, but they often come in a petrochemical base or are synthetically derived. Use of over-the-counter preparations to eliminate lice should be evaluated on an individual basis.

❖ MEASLES ❖

Rubeola, or "ten-day measles," was considered a common childhood illness prior to the advent of vaccinations. Sometimes it became a complicated illness, especially in those malnourished or already ill, but many people experienced it and came through just fine. The vaccine has decreased the illness's incidence; however, vaccination does not guarantee lifelong immunity. The illness itself, interestingly enough, usually does confer lifelong resistance to the disease.

Owing to the recent resurgence of measles and the virulence of the strain associated with it, there has been some degree of measles hysteria that has blown its risk out of proportion. While serious nervous system and other reactions to measles have been repeatedly reported in the medical literature, they are based on the worst and rarest scenarios of the disease: brain damage, encephalitis, muscle paralysis, and blindness. Other risks and complications associated with measles include pneumonia, ear infections, and lymph-node infections. These are all rare and generally preventable.

Traditional practitioners, particularly those trained in Eastern medicine, regard measles as a strengthening and purifying illness, one not to be suppressed or discouraged. For example, according to Bob Flaws (1985), "Chinese medicine believes that measles are not just an infectious epidemic disease but rather a symptom of a preexisting internal disharmony." Dietary, environmental, and other "poisons" the child accumulates from even before birth create heat in the body that then allows the measles to manifest. According to this philosophy, the body's effort to eliminate and discharge the heat should be encouraged and supported.

Measles begins like a cold with a runny nose, cough, fever, and general achiness. Sometimes the eyes are sore or sensitive to light. Little white spots on the inside of the mouth ("Kopliks spots") that are characteristic of measles may occur but are not always noticed. The fever tends to get progressively higher, often reaching between 103 and 105 degrees Fahrenheit on the third or fourth day. By this time a rash will begin to appear, probably around the hairline of the head, behind the ears, on the neck or face. During this eruptive phase the child will probably feel the worst. Though the rash is not itchy, the child will probably have no appetite, have a sore throat or cough, and diarrhea, and may feel listless. This stage lasts for a few days until the rash is fully developed, at which time the symptoms, including the fever, begin to subside. After another week or so the rash fades.

Measles are contagious starting about five days after exposure to the virus and until about ten days after the rash first appears. It is airborne, being spread by sneezing and coughing and through contact with the sick person's mucus. The incubation period (the time between exposure and appearance of symptoms) is about ten to fifteen days. Spring may be the most likely time to see this illness.

WHEN TO SEEK MEDICAL CARE

Seek a skilled opinion and medical care if the child is very young, or if you feel uncomfortable with home care; if the child's high fever persists even after the rash has fully appeared; if your child develops chest pain, breathing difficulty, or severe cough; if your child has seizures or severe headache, loses consciousness, acts delirious, or has a stiff neck; if your child develops a severe earache that does not respond to basic earache treatment.

Complications of measles are rare in healthy kids, but it is best to be aware of them so you can seek help quickly should your child require it.

CARING FOR THE CHILD WITH MEASLES

It is imperative that you keep your child at home and restful from the time you know of exposure (begin treatment then) or begin to see symptoms and until a week or so after the rash begins to fade. This will allow time for optimal nourishment, which can prevent complications and allow maximum benefit from the illness while ensuring complete recovery of strength. Keeping the child home for the duration also limits exposure of others to measles.

If other family members have not had the illness themselves, keeping them home from school and other public places for ten days may be best because they also may be carriers.

- During the first phase of measles, when your child is just beginning to feel ill, bedrest and general comfort measures for symptoms are in order (refer to other sections in this chapter—"Fevers" and "Achiness," for example).

- Throughout the illness frequently provide your child with your choice of the following infusions: elder blossom, peppermint, and calendula; or lemon balm, catnip, licorice root, elder flowers, and violet leaves; or burdock root and peppermint; or yarrow and lemon balm.

  Choose the herbs you want to use and mix up a batch in roughly equal parts. Take a handful of the mix and steep in a covered quart jar of boiling water for twenty minutes. (Burdock root must be steeped for two hours.) Strain and sweeten to taste with honey or maple syrup. Give frequently, up to 2 quarts a day, as hot as can be tolerated to encourage sweating. You can recombine these herbs any way you like.

  These infusions help relieve discomforts while opening the pores to discharge heat, bring on the rash, and facilitate the next phases. The herbs suggested combine several properties: they are diaphoretic (they increase or induce perspiration), alterative (health restoring), relaxant, and soothing to upset stomachs, feverishness, and irritability.

- Give echinacea tincture, 1 drop per 2 pounds of body weight four times a day. This supports your child's immune system while he or she is processing the infection, preventing secondary infections. Along with echinacea, 10 to 30 drops of astragalus tincture three times daily assists the immune system and the skin as well.

- Chamomile tea can be given to soothe the nerves and tummy.

- Diet during fevers should be as light as possible. When the child feels hungry, give soup, seasonal fruits, steamed vegetables, and soupy grains.

- Give plenty of fluids, especially water and tea, throughout the illness to flush the system and prevent dehydration. The child should drink some fluids every waking hour. Avoid orange juice.

- For sore eyes, apply compresses of chamomile or eyebright as described in "Conjunctivitis." Keep the child's room dark to prevent eye discomforts.
- Coughs may accompany measles. To ease coughing and prevent stagnation of mucus which harbors infection and could lead to pneumonia, study the section on coughs and provide appropriate remedies.
- Warm baths, no more than a couple of degrees cooler than body temperature, may be given as a comfort measure to very feverish children. Calendula, thyme, marshmallow root, burdock root, chickweed, lemon balm, plantain, and gingerroot are all excellent choices for an herbal bath. They can be used alone or in combination to ease fever and skin irritation and to draw out the infection. Add a strong infusion of 2 ounces of herbs and 2 quarts of water, steeped for one hour to the bathwater. Be sure to avoid letting the child get chilled when getting out of the tub.

DURING RECOVERY

- Continue to use echinacea tincture until the child seems strong. Gradually decrease the dosage and frequency until you are giving just 1 drop per 5 pounds of body weight twice a day.
- Feed your child nutritious foods but continue to limit dairy, meat, sugar, and refined or processed foods for some time. Porridges and hearty soups are wonderful.
- Dandelion or agrimony can stimulate a slow appetite back to health. You can use infusions, but these herbs are bitter; tinctures are easier to swallow. Dosage is 10 to 20 drops of either a few times a day.
- Provide kudzu-apple juice (see "Colds and Flu"), miso broth (preferably with shiitake mushrooms), slippery elm bark tea, or marshmallow root tea to rebuild fluid lost during the fever. These preparations are traditionally used for convalescence. Add honey and cinnamon to flavor the teas and make them more tonifying.
- Encourage your child to slowly and gently resume activities. There's no need to rush him back to school or social activities. Having your child recuperate for as long as he was ill, providing slightly more fresh air and gentle exercise each day that he is up to it, may be wise.

❖ MENINGITIS ❖

Bacterial meningitis is the inflammation of the meninges, the tissue covering the brain and spinal cord, and is caused by a bacterial infection. It can occur at any age and fortunately is relatively rare. Meningitis can quickly lead to severe retardation and death.

WHEN TO SEEK MEDICAL CARE

IF YOU SUSPECT MENINGITIS, SEEK IMMEDIATE MEDICAL CARE. Common signs of meningitis are fever or subnormal temperature, stiffness or soreness of the neck when the child is asked to place her chin on her chest, vomiting, poor feeding, inconsolable crying (which is sometimes high pitched), irritability, headache (often severe), not wanting to be held, discomfort when the legs are raised toward the chest (as when changing diapers or when the child is put into a similar knees-to-chest position lying on the back), sensitivity to light, unusual rash (especially in older children or adults), and, in babies, a bulging fontanel (the soft spot on the head). Someone with meningitis can exhibit any of these symptoms, but the disease can be subtle and appear to be just a general illness. Insist that your child be thoroughly evaluated and checked for meningitis if you suspect that it may be the problem.

Antibiotic therapy is the most practical approach to meningitis because it is quick acting and readily available. Natural healing can be used with the antibiotics and afterward to promote thorough recovery. Quick treatment usually offers the very best opportunity for a positive outcome.

Meningitis can occur unexpectedly but often as a complication of an already-existing illness (such as measles). It may occur in conjunction with travels to foreign countries where the disease is more prevalent. I've noticed that epidemics often break out in the heat of summer, but the disease can appear at any time of the year. Macrobiotic teachings emphasize that excessive consumption of certain foods that are considered "yin" or cold in nature, such as juices, fruits, or ice cream, create a ripe condition for meningitis. Interestingly enough, kids do tend to consume more than usual amounts of these foods in the summer. Epidemics also occur when kids have been in the same public swimming pool as someone with the bacteria.

I offer no suggestions for treatment here. Prompt medical intervention is absolutely appropriate for meningitis. Please bear in mind that while the consequences of meningitis can be devastating, not all fevers, headaches, or vomiting mean that your child has this illness. Using the above list of symptoms as a guide, observe your child carefully, and if you have sufficient concern, check it out.

❖ MUMPS ❖

Mumps, another of the many viral infections common to childhood, is a swelling of the parotid glands (salivary glands), located on the jaw line just below and in front of the earlobe. The incubation period is two to three weeks, after which the child feels mildly ill and the parotid glands on one side of the face begin swelling. The area can become so swollen that the cheek and neck seem quite thick. The swelling may then begin to appear on the other side of the cheek as well. The child often experiences fever, malaise, and pain behind the ear when chewing or swallowing. It is contagious from the day before the swelling appears until the swelling is gone, usually a week to ten days later.

Mumps frequently occurs before ten years of age and confers lifelong immunity. Occasionally it leads to swollen testicles in pubescent boys; very rarely girls of this age develop swollen ovaries. This hardly ever leads to problems of sterility and usually affects only one gonad or the other.

WHEN TO SEEK MEDICAL CARE

Encephalitis, though unlikely, is a possible complication of mumps that parents should be aware of. Symptoms include sudden and extreme rise in fever, neck or back stiffness, sudden severe headache, projectile vomiting, and mental fogginess. Seek medical care if any of these signs arise.

GENERAL RECOMMENDATIONS

- Provide your child with a comfortable resting place with plenty of simple activities and stories to keep him occupied and distracted from his discomfort.
- Your child should drink plenty of fluids frequently, especially in the case of fever. Provide straws to make drinking easier.
- Give foods that are easy to swallow, easy to digest, and completely natural. Giving ice cream, yogurt, or other cool and creamy foods may be tempting, but they are not beneficial. Rather, give soups, teas, freshly prepared fruit and vegetable juices, blended or stewed fruits, steamed vegetables, and porridges such as cream of rice.

HERBAL RECOMMENDATIONS

These remedies in combination have a gentle but definite ability to reduce inflammation in the glands:

- A tincture combining burdock root, dandelion root, and chick-weed in equal parts should be given in a dose of 10 to 40 drops four times a day.
- In addition, give 20 drops of echinacea tincture and 500 milli-grams of vitamin C four times a day.
- You can also have your child drink infusions of any of the following herbs, alone or in combination, throughout the day to enhance healing: red clover blossoms, calendula, cleavers, chamomile, catnip, and thyme.
- Garlic lemonade and kudzu-apple juice (see "Colds and Flu") may also be taken freely.
- Externally apply compresses to reduce the swelling and pain. Par-ticularly useful are infusions of violet leaves, calendula, and cha-momile. A hot-water bottle can provide additional relief.
- Refer also to the section on fevers.

❖ NIGHTMARES AND SLEEP DISTURBANCES ❖

Children are impressionable. If your child is having nightmares, some-thing she saw or heard has likely disturbed her. Be supportive and com-forting as you encourage your child to talk about what is frightening her. Listen without judgment: what may seem silly to you may be terrifying to a child. Rather than just saying, "That's silly and nothing to be afraid of," help the child understand or overcome the fear. Often telling a short story in which the child is the hero can help him or her resolve the issue.

Television and movie images are major culprits of nightmares. The only time my son has ever had a nightmare was when he was two and saw *Sesame Street* for the first time. Most kids are watching programs that are much more violent and serious than this. Limiting what your child views can relieve nightmares.

Children also experience stress in their lives. If your child is having persistent nightmares and you are unable to determine their source but suspect a problem at home or school is causing them, an experienced counselor may be able to help.

A child who has had a nightmare often gets to spend the rest of the night in the parental bed. Perhaps the nightmares are a vehicle for gain-ing this privilege. Consider the possibility that your child really wants to be near you at night, and contemplate arranging a family bed or at least a family bedroom for a while. Actually, most people in the world sleep in one room, often in one bed. You can read about this idea in Tine Thevenin's book *The Family Bed: An Age Old Concept in Child Rearing* (see "Further Reading").

In any case, you can make bedtime special by creating rituals that help your child go to sleep feeling secure. A consistent bedtime, perhaps a lit candle or soft lamp, lots of love and cuddles, a peaceful story, and a song will help almost any child let go of the day's worries and embrace sleep. You can even hold your child's hand until he has fallen asleep. Your child will appreciate the time you share with him. Be sure to blow out any lit candles before leaving the child's room.

Foods that are eaten too close to bedtime can cause digestive up-sets that hinder the child from falling asleep and contribute to sleep disturbances. Heavy meals, spicy foods, and sweets are especially stimu-lating, so certainly avoid these. Eat supper at least two hours before bedtime. If supper is running late, prepare something easy to digest. A small portion of yogurt (at room temperature), a cup of warm milk with a pinch of cinnamon and honey, or a cup of warm almond milk (also with cinnamon and honey) are all pleasant-tasting and sleep-promoting bedtime beverages.

Pinworms can cause periodic restlessness during sleep. Teething and earaches can cause sleeping difficulties. Your child may also exhibit sleep-ing problems on a cyclical basis, usually for a few nights in a row, every two weeks or monthly. In these cases, the child will often wake up a few times during the night whimpering or crying but can often be comforted back to sleep with earache or teething remedies and rocking. Pinworms cause restlessness, not easily resolvable with comfort. Of course, any underlying causes need to be addressed directly in order for the problem to be solved, so refer to "Intestinal Parasites" or "Earaches and Ear In-fections" in this chapter, or "Teething" in Chapter 7 for information on those conditions.

Herbal Recommendations

- Particularly beneficial herbs and formulas include Calm Child Formula (see "Car Sickness"), Mother's Milk Tea II (see "Colic [or the Sunset Blues]" in Chapter 7), chamomile, catnip, lemon balm, lime blossom, lavender, and hops. Prepare as standard teas and administer on a daily basis to tonify the nervous system. Hops, the herb used in beer making, is frequently used to encourage a restful sleep. If your child is anxious, 10 drops of tincture can be given in 1/4 cup warm water at bedtime to help her relax.
- Herbal pillows, sometimes called "dream pillows," are a wonderful gift for any child, especially those who have difficulty sleeping through the night. An herbal pillow is simple to prepare and can be done with your child. It is generally small—for example, a rectangle

about 10 inches by 12 inches or another shape approximately equivalent in size. It can be in a basic shape or cut in the form of a moon, star, cat, heart, whatever.

You need to make an outer covering and an inner pillow that will enclose the herbs. Muslin is a good choice for the inner pillow because it will keep the herbs from prickling your child's face or sifting through the fabric as they get ground down over time. Stuff the pillow full with lavender, chamomile, rosemary, hops, mugwort, or catnip.

- Prior to bedtime try giving your child an herbal bath using a few drops of essential oils or infusions of chamomile, lavender, rose, lemon grass, or other calming herbs.

❖ Nosebleeds ❖

Usually you can stop a nosebleed by having the child sit calmly while you hold the nostrils closed with pressure from the thumb and index finger. This encourages clotting. After a few minutes, release the fingers to see if the bleeding has stopped. If not, apply pressure again with the head tilted back. In addition, a cool cloth can be applied to the nape of the neck.

WHEN TO SEEK MEDICAL CARE

Nosebleeds are not dangerous unless the bleeding is unstoppable. Any nosebleed that occurs after a severe head injury or is uncontrollable requires further attention.

GENERAL RECOMMENDATIONS

- Witch hazel (the herb or the extract), calendula, bayberry bark, white oak bark, and yarrow are astringents recognized for their ability to stop bleeding. To use, make an infusion and soak some tissue or a piece of cotton ball in it, and insert into the nostril. Alternatively, some of the powdered herb can be sprinkled into or snuffed up the nostril.
- Human hair is an old remedy for many kinds of hemorrhages and is employed in the traditional medicines of many cultures. A small amount of hair is burned to ash in a small dish and used just like the powdered herbs mentioned above. It may sound strange, but if you haven't any other herbs on hand, you can use hair instead. For a nosebleed it takes only a tiny bit.

- Dry air from winter heating can aggravate the tendency to get nosebleeds, so run a humidifier in your child's room or find an alternative method of moistening the air.
- Chronic nosebleeds require that you do more than first-aid. A child with this condition needs an herbal program addressing constitutional imbalance. Herbs that strengthen the circulatory system, such as nettles, raspberry leaf, buckwheat, black currants, yellow dock, and motherwort, can be given regularly for this purpose. A diet rich in greens and whole grains and deemphasizing sweets and cold foods also helps prevent nosebleeds.

❖ PENIS IRRITATIONS AND CARE ❖

Up to about three or four years old, little boys who are uncircumcised need not give much more thought to genital hygiene than they do to belly-button hygiene. When you bathe your son, gently wash his whole body with a wash cloth and soap. Retracting the foreskin is unnecessary; the glands do not secrete much oil so there won't be any buildup of secretions. *Smegma*, which in Greek actually means "soap," is the name of the oil that is secreted as your child matures.

Forcible retraction of the foreskin can cause adhesions of the skin that can cause retraction problems later. The normal "fiddling" around that your child does with his penis is sufficient to encourage normal retractability. It is healthy and fine to let a child play with himself. You can talk to him about appropriate times and places if you have a toddler with an exhibitionist streak or prudish grandparents!

At about age four the glands become more active, at which time you can teach your son to *gently* pull the foreskin back a little to clean out any accumulated discharge. This can simply be part of regular bathing. In warmer weather he can be do it daily or every couple of days, again as just part of regular bathing.

GENERAL RECOMMENDATIONS

Stress, extreme heat and humidity, and lapses in hygiene may lead to a buildup of discharge that can cause irritation or even a small abscess. Treat as follows:

- Wash the penis well with warm water, loosening and cleaning away any pus or discharge. Do this twice a day.
- Apply either calendula oil or healing salve after each wash. Aloe vera gel is also antiseptic, healing, and soothing.

- Let the child soak in the tub if he is uncomfortable. Herbs such as lavender, thyme, calendula, garlic, uva ursi, or rosemary can be added in infusion or oil form. Or add 1 cup of sea salt per bath.

Internally give the following:

- Plenty of water to encourage the area to be flushed naturally during urination
- Echinacea tincture, 15 to 30 drops four times a day
- 500 milligrams of vitamin C four times daily

You should notice some improvement within twenty-four hours. Refer to "Abscesses" and see a physician if necessary.

If your son is complaining of burning upon urination, he could have a urinary-tract infection. Refer to that section for information.

❖ Poison Ivy and Poison Oak ❖

Poison ivy (*Rhus toxicodendron*) is a common plant with characteristic "leaves of three." It can be a low-growing plant, a climbing vine, or an erect shrub. Consult a field guide so that you can recognize it. Contact with the plant's oil can cause extremely itchy dermatitis. The outbreak may not occur for several hours, or even several days, after contact with the plant.

Poison oak (*Rhus radicans* or *R. diversiloba*) is closely related to poison ivy, having the same active oil. Symptoms are similar and treatment is the same.

Susceptibility to the oil of these plants varies from person to person, and even within the same person. In fact, I've touched poison ivy many times without ever having a reaction—until a few days ago when I weeded our garden—so these remedies are especially close to my heart (and left arm) at the moment!

Symptoms are a small rash that itches intensely or may burn. If your child avoids scratching the rash, the outbreak remains localized and heals more quickly than if she scratches it. The rash sometimes turns into small fluid-filled blisters, which may weep and then crust over. Symptoms can persist for days, but outbreaks have been known to last for weeks or more.

General Recommendations

- Upon contact, thoroughly wash the area as soon as possible with soap and water. This will remove, as much as possible, the volatile oils on the skin.

- Next apply lotions, washes, or pastes of jewel weed, calendula, plantain, green clay, or apple cider vinegar. These help reduce inflammation and prevent extreme itchiness. Either marshmallow root or slippery elm bark in powder form can be made into a paste and applied alternately with the aforementioned herbs to prevent dryness and chafing of the skin. Tea tree oil can be used to reduce itching and dry up the rash.
- Taken internally, tinctures or infusions of any of the following herbs can also reduce inflammation and discomfort: echinacea, burdock root, chickweed, plantain, calendula, slippery elm, marshmallow root.
- All of the herbs mentioned can also be used in tincture form. If you plan to be in an area with a lot of poison ivy or oak, it may be wise to carry a selection of these tinctures with you. In addition, carry some healing salve.
- At home, a bath with any of the above herbs, apple cider vinegar, or baking soda can relieve itching.
- *Rhus tox.* 30x, a homeopathic preparation of poison ivy, is indicated. Give it repeatedly as necessary.
- Guide your child through a visualization (see "Asthma") to help him get comfortable and rest.
- The rash's itching is likely to make your child very uncomfortable. Herbs listed in the sections on irritability and nightmares are excellent for helping him relax.

❖ RINGWORM ❖

Ringworm is not a worm but a fungal infection. Athlete's foot is caused by the same fungus. Ringworm is characterized by a raised ring of tiny scales surrounding normal-looking skin. There may be one patch or many; the patches may be large or small. Ringworm is not dangerous though it may itch and it is a nuisance. On the scalp it can cause temporary hair loss in the affected areas.

Ringworm is highly contagious and spread by contact with an infected person or pet or even with infected clothing, linens, shower floors, and the like. To avoid its spread and reinfection, observe scrupulous hygiene and isolate the personal items of the affected person. Wash all clothes and linens in a hot-water wash cycle every couple of days.

HERBAL RECOMMENDATIONS

A one-time infection of ringworm should readily respond to external treatments that destroy the fungus and strengthen the skin's natural antimicrobial functions. Choose one or two remedies from the suggestions below. Treatment may require from a few days to more than a week to be completely effective. Repeating applications two to three times a day and using strong infusions for washes or full-strength tinctures are important. Cotton balls make the best applicators for tinctures and oils. Discard them immediately after each use. Once an applicator touches the skin, it should not touch anything else.

Repeated bouts of ringworm may indicate that the body is not functioning optimally to resist infection and that hygiene may not be adequate. You will want to take herbal and dietary measures to promote immune-system health in addition to the recommendations that follow and to pay extra-close attention to cleanliness. For the treatment of chronic skin parasites, read the information about immunity in "Rashes and Skin Problems."

- Black walnut is one of the most widely respected antifungals of the herbal world. Black walnut trees are found abundantly in North America. The hulls are rich in an orange-brown liquid that is a natural source of iodine, which is used medically as a topical antiseptic. The hulls, leaves, and bark of the plant can be used. Tincture of black walnut is probably the easiest preparation to use. Apply liberally and let dry. Any discoloration of the skin is temporary.
- Essential oils of lavender, rosemary, or thyme are effective against ringworm. They may be applied directly or diluted in a small amount of vegetable oil in a proportion of 1:1. Dilution is best for sensitive skin. Do not apply essential oils near the eyes as they are too caustic, just on the affected area and immediately around it.
- The following antiparasite wash is very helpful for skin infections. Mix 3 ounces apple cider vinegar; 2 teaspoons each of calendula oil and goldenseal tincture; and 1 teaspoon each of thyme oil, lavender oil, and myrrh powder. Store in a glass bottle, labeled with the contents, the date, and the warning FOR EXTERNAL USE ONLY. Shake well before each use, apply liberally, and let dry. This preparation will keep for years if stored in a cool, dark place.
- St. John's wort is considered to have antifungal properties and may be used for ringworm. Apply the oil extract to the affected areas two to three times a day.

❖ SCABIES ❖

Scabies are little mites, or body lice, that burrow in the skin where they then lay their eggs. They cause intense itching, especially at night. An initial infestation may incubate for up to three weeks. Reinfestation is usually noticed within two days because the body has become highly sensitized. Scabies are spread by physical contact. They are often spread to people by household pets. Exposure to scabies does not necessarily mean that an infection will occur, however. For example, when my son was seven he spent the night at the home of a family who unknowingly had scabies, but my son did not pick them up. As soon as we knew of the family's condition, we used preventive herbal treatments.

GENERAL RECOMMENDATIONS

Conventional treatment for scabies includes meticulous housecleaning and the external use of strong chemical preparations. Natural treatment requires the same intense diligence with housecleaning and the use of personal hygiene and herbs.

- Scabies can be a challenge to eliminate, especially because the itching may persist for days after they are dead. This leaves you unsure as to whether the treatment was effective or if scabies are still present. Maintain treatment for seven days; then repeat for two days in each of two additional consecutive weeks. This will help ensure that new mites are killed at the beginning of their life cycle and prevent reinfection.
- Change clothing daily. Wash all laundry and clean rugs and furnishings every two to three days. Wash all clothing, towels, and linens in the hot wash cycle. Since scabies can live on furniture cushions, you may want to limit use of some chairs and sofas until the infestation has passed, and cover the furniture in use with sheets, blankets, or other coverings. These will be easier to launder than the cushions themselves. This level of housecleaning can be draining and exhausting but must be done to ensure that reinfestation does not occur.
- In extremely cold climates, consider vacating your home and leaving it unheated for two to three days, freezing the scabies and denying them a host. The temperature must stay below 30 degrees Fahrenheit in the house. This, however, is not a guaranteed solution.
- Quarantine and treat all pets. Speak with your veterinarian about the options.

HERBAL RECOMMENDATIONS

- Give a daily hot bath with "Green Soap," which is available at some pharmacies (frequently the older ones carry it) or undiluted Dr. Bronner's liquid Castile soap. Use the peppermint- or lavender-scented soap for optimal effectiveness; these herbs reduce parasite infestations. Gently scrubbing the skin with a stiff brush such as a back scrubber helps open the pores and allows the soap and herbs to penetrate the skin.

- After the bath, apply the antiparasite wash described in "Ringworm," adding an extra tablespoon of lavender oil to the recipe. The wash should be applied liberally all over the body.
- For repeated infestations, try getting your family to eat a lot of garlic—cloves, tea, or capsules—along with the above remedies. Garlic is a strong-smelling herb and is considered a natural insecticide. It is also specifically useful for strengthening the body's resistance to parasites.
- If you choose to use a prescription substance, use one such as Elimite, which is prepared from pyrethrins, plant-based insecticides. DO NOT USE KWELL: It is too dangerous to apply to the whole body, especially for young children.

❖ Skin Problems (General) ❖

The skin is a huge organ of communication and protection. Covering us from head to toe, it is, so to speak, our interface with the world around us. Through our skin we regulate our body temperature and resist external elements like water, germs, and heat; and through our many nerve endings we experience and share both pain and pleasure. The skin is also a major organ of elimination. Through it we discharge old cells, waste products, and illnesses.

Rashes and skin problems (eczema, psoriasis, and allergies) are a reflection of either internal processes that need attention or the body's effort to resist external irritants. By viewing ourselves and our children as perfect organisms, we can approach the skin's symptoms as messages rather than problems.

Immunity, Digestion, and the Skin's Health

If the skin is sending messages, listen to them. Are there other messages as well? For example, is your child always chilly, and does she often get sick? Perhaps her resistance is low and needs to be strengthened. Is there constipation? kidney weakness? Because the skin is a major organ of resistance, building immune-system health also helps the skin. Once or twice a week, give your child soup made from broth in which the following herbs have been cooked for thirty minutes. Per 2 quarts of water include four shiitake mushrooms, two pieces of astragalus root, 1 teaspoon red ginseng root, and four to six pieces of codonopsis. Vegetable or chicken stock make good bases for this herbal tonic soup.

These herbs, which originate in China but can also be found in the United States, are traditionally used to enhance the "Wei Chi," the body's ability to resist illness and susceptibility. The Wei Chi resides at the skin and in the lungs. Interestingly, the use of steroids is related to both asthma and skin complaints, both in treatment and in side effects. Other herbs that specifically enhance resistance to infection are garlic, calendula, and echinacea.

When the body's ability to eliminate waste through the bowels and bladder is weak or blocked, the skin will assist in that function and as a result may show stress. Acne, pimples, and eczema may all be reflections of the skin being overtaxed as it compensates for the other eliminatory organs trying to eliminate the wastes accumulating in the body. Refer to "Constipation" and "Urinary-Tract Infections" to strengthen the bowels and urinary organs if this seems to be an underlying cause of your child's skin troubles.

An unhealthy diet loaded with chemicals, additives, oils, and processed foods only adds to the skin's burden. Similarly, a food that causes an allergy forces the body to try to rapidly eliminate that substance and may tax the skin, leading to hives, rashes, and itching. Replacing an allergen in the diet until the child can tolerate it usually reduces the skin complaint. To identify allergens (which may not just be foods but can include household products, certain fabrics, and other things), pay attention to what a child has done or eaten within twenty-four hours of the reaction. Perhaps an obvious pattern will emerge. Local irritants such as a wet diaper or tight-fitting sneakers can cause a skin reaction such as diaper rash or blisters. Try to remove any obvious causes of a skin problem and apply the appropriate remedy.

Stress undermines our well-being, as does a lack of communication within our relationships. Because the skin is our interface with the world, stress, anxiety, anger, and fear can manifest in skin symptoms. As with allergies, closely observe your children to detect any correlations between certain experiences and skin reactions. Help them learn to reduce stress in their lives and to communicate in some way (verbally, artistically, in a journal, and so forth) rather than internalizing their feelings. Channeling their energy in positive ways will establish an important life-long precedent that cannot be overvalued.

Herbal Recommendations

The recommendations that follow are "skin foods," herbs that nourish and heal the skin. For specific conditions, see other sections such as

"Acne" and "Abscesses." In "Acne" you will find detailed dietary information useful for addressing most skin complaints.

- My favorite herbs used internally for skin eruptions include burdock root, echinacea, calendula, nettles, chickweed, dandelion root, red clover, yellow dock, violet leaves, plantain, and astragalus. Use standard infusions or tinctures of these herbs, either alone or in combination.
- External preparations for healing the skin can be in the form of salves, powders, washes, baths, poultices, and compresses. For dry skin, scrapes, bites, and itches, I prefer salves. For runny or wet-looking sores, powders work nicely. They absorb drainage while providing protection and often antiseptic and healing-promoting properties to the sore. Hot compresses, poultices, and soaks are excellent for infections, and baths are soothing for all-over rashes and itches such as those from poison ivy and chickenpox. Favorites include all the herbs mentioned for internal use, plus slippery elm bark, marshmallow root, myrrh, lavender, chaparral, green clay, and apple cider vinegar. Raw honey can be applied directly to pimples, scrapes, and cuts. It is drawing and antiseptic.

❖ SORE THROAT ❖

A variety of factors can cause a sore throat. Fatigue, dry air from heat sources in the winter, too much heat or dryness in the body (which many times is also a result of exhaustion), viral or bacterial infection, even suppressed anger—all can lead up to that scratchy, sometimes painful feeling. A sore throat may herald a cold or upper respiratory infection. A strep infection (discussed later in this section) often causes an extremely sore throat.

PREVENTION

- Insist that your child get plenty of rest. Fatigue is one of the biggest causes of lowered resistance in both children and adults.
- Place a pot of hot water on your heater if possible to do so safely (on a wood stove, for example) or run a humidifier to moisten the air on winter nights.
- Allow your child to express his or her feelings, including anger.
- When winter changes into spring, provide a slightly lighter diet. Adding fresh greens and cutting back on heavy foods will assist the body's inner temperature to adjust to the seasonal change. Likewise, in autumn, cut back on cold-natured foods and add

more warming and hearty foods. Being in harmony with the seasons not only heightens our awareness of the natural world but also increases our likelihood of staying well.

- Attend to infections as soon as they arise to prevent them from worsening.

HERBAL RECOMMENDATIONS

- For sore throat associated with fever, strep, or other inflammatory process, you will want to provide herbs that mildly cool and bring moisture to the body. Burdock root, dandelion root, or chickweed tincture, alone or in combination, may be used for this purpose. Dosage is 1 dropperful of tincture or infusion applied directly on the throat by eyedropper or spray (using a bottle with a small mister on top) or by sipping or gargling. The tincture should be first diluted in a couple tablespoons of warm water. Repeat as needed.

- Mucilaginous herbs provide moisture and soothing coolness to the throat while addressing heat and dryness in the system. Examples of these herbs are marshmallow root, slippery elm bark, comfrey root, Irish moss, and kudzu root (see "Colds and Flu"). These herbs should be taken as standard infusions. You can give kudzu in kudzu-apple juice (also under "Colds and Flu"), and slippery elm can be made into lozenges. See "Herbal Preparations" in Chapter 4 for directions on making lozenges.

- A tea combining slippery elm and cinnamon makes a delicious and soothing drink for sore throats accompanying colds and clear runny noses, loose bowels, chills, or other signs of a cold. It warms the circulation, provides moisture to the throat, and strengthens the bowels while preventing the griping associated with diarrhea. It can be taken any time for general well-being and is an excellent winter-time beverage. To prepare, stir 1 teaspoon slippery elm bark powder and 1/2 teaspoon cinnamon powder into 1 cup boiling water. Stir very well, steep for five minutes, and sweeten with honey. Serve warm.

- Honey, lemon, and ginger can be taken by the teaspoon to soothe a sore throat and to prevent infections from worsening. Mix 1/2 teaspoon of honey with equal parts of lemon juice and freshly squeezed ginger juice. To make ginger juice, grate a 1-inch piece of fresh ginger root and squeeze the gratings. One clove of freshly chopped garlic can replace the ginger.

- For comfort your child can gargle with or sip thyme tea with honey or sweetened sage tea (sage is not safe during pregnancy); sip garlic lemonade (see "Colds or Flu"); or drink large amounts of catnip and lemon balm tea. Use as needed.

- To reduce inflammation and infection in the throat, have your child gargle a mixture of 1/2 cup warm water, 1/2 teaspoon good-quality sea salt, and 1/2 teaspoon myrrh powder.
- In addition to any of the above choices, give your child 10 to 50 drops of echinacea tincture and 250 to 1,000 milligrams of vitamin C depending on the age of the child, every four hours.

❖ STREP THROAT ❖

Strep throat, caused by a proliferation of Group A beta-hemolytic streptococcus bacteria, is characterized by deep fatigue or malaise, generally a very sore throat, and fever, which may be as high as 104 degrees Fahrenheit. The back of the throat usually exhibits visible spots of pus. To see these, have your child open his mouth and say "Ahhhh" while standing in good light. Although the illness is not generally serious, the person will feel extremely ill. A person with a weakened immune system or prior kidney problems, or one in whom the illness goes completely untreated, runs the risk of developing complications.

Strep is a common response to exhaustion (the deeper cause of the illness) and, consequently, to lowered immunity. It can be successfully treated at home, but the child must be closely monitored to see that the infection is improving. Although rare, rheumatic fever and kidney infection can be serious complications of the illness.

WHEN TO SEEK MEDICAL CARE

If you don't see some improvement in two days, or if you see any worsening, medical attention is justified. The assistance of a physician is warranted for strep occurring in very young children (under two years). Testing for strep at the doctor's office merely involves taking a culture of the bacteria from the throat. Antibiotics are the usual medical treatment. As with all fevers and infections, dehydration must be prevented with plentiful fluid intake.

In addition to the general herbal remedies for sore throat:

- Give echinacea and vitamin C as often as specified above, but on the higher side, giving 1 drop of echinacea for every 2 pounds of your child's body weight.
- Along with these, give 3 to 20 drops (according to age) of goldenseal tincture.

- Give 4 to 6 tablets of alfalfa every four hours and plentiful amounts of water. If you can't find alfalfa tablets or if the child is too young to swallow them, give liquid chlorophyll, which is easy to disguise in other beverages.
- A light diet of warm teas and broth is advisable.
- Raw garlic is a must. You can mince a clove and put it into a teaspoon of honey, making it easy to swallow, or you can make a garlic-and-honey syrup by blending the two together with enough honey to make it palatable (but not overly diluted—it should still be spicy). Give the child the equivalent of a clove of garlic every few hours. Chase the spicy taste with a piece of raw apple or a few sips of unfiltered apple juice.

❖ STOMACH ACHES ❖

Few kids get through childhood without at least one stomach ache. Stomach aches most often occur when a child is overwhelmed, nervous, tired, or, of course, eats too much "birthday-party" food. Anxiety frequently experienced en route to a test at school or the dentist's office, for example, can give kids that nauseous, fluttery feeling known as "butterflies." A full bladder, gas, hunger, or constipation can also lead to this complaint.

Other common conditions that can cause stomach aches are intestinal parasites and urinary-tract infections. You can refer to those headings for further information.

WHEN TO SEEK MEDICAL CARE

A sudden, acute "stomach ache" that occurs on the lower right side of the abdomen may be appendicitis. If there is great tenderness and other symptoms such as nausea, fever, diarrhea, and bad breath, seek medical help.

GENERAL RECOMMENDATIONS

- Encourage your child to use the bathroom and take some time to relax. Talk with the child about any anxieties that may be on her mind. Frequently these simple measures will do the trick. Sometimes all we have to do is really listen to what our children are trying to tell us.
- A cup of warm tea can provide a relaxing focus for you and your child. Many herbs are favored for stomach ills.

- Rubbing your child's tummy, even with a simple oil massage, can be quite comforting. Your child will need your quiet reassurance and understanding if anxiety is at the root of the discomfort.

HERBAL RECOMMENDATIONS

- These tummy teas are well respected for their ability to eliminate stomach aches from simple causes such as gas, anxiety, and indigestion: chamomile, lemon balm, catnip, fennel seed, anise seed, peppermint, ginger root, spearmint, kudzu root. They can be used alone or in a variety of tasty combinations. Be creative!
- Mother's Milk Tea II really is as soothing as mother's milk! Perfect for a stomach ache, it is immediately calming and delicious, and it is an excellent expeller of intestinal gas. See "Colic (or the Sunset Blues)" in Chapter 7 for the recipe. It can be taken as often as needed until the complaint has passed.
- You can give activated charcoal powder if the child has a very uncomfortable stomach ache from overeating, if there's lots of belching, or if the cause of the ache is just simple indigestion. Give in capsules or pills, or, if the child is unable to swallow them, give 1/4 teaspoon of the powder dissolved in 2 tablespoons warm water. Repeat in a half hour if necessary.
- For babies with tummy trouble, see "Colic (or the Sunset Blues)" in Chapter 7.

❖ STYES ❖

Styes are localized bacterial infections that occur around the eye, on the rim of the upper or lower lid, and often along the base of an eyelash. They are generally small and harmless but can cause intense itching or discomfort. They may develop along with conjunctivitis, or conjunctivitis may develop as a secondary infection as a result of the child rubbing his eyes a lot from the irritation.

Styes can be a result of local irritation, such as a piece of sand or an eyelash, but they are also the body's way of eliminating accumulated waste, particularly if other eliminatory avenues are not working optimally. Therefore, if your child is prone to styes, look toward strengthening his or her elimination system (refer to "Bed-Wetting," "Constipation," "Skin Problems [General]," and "Urinary-Tract Infections"). Also be sure that your kid is getting plenty of fluids. Styes are pretty easy to clear up with simple home treatment.

General Recommendations

- Reduce the amount of fat, dairy, and flour products in the diet. They increase the body's production of mucus and therefore the amount of discharge.
- Give your child more fresh fruits and vegetables. If possible, give your child freshly made carrot juice. A wonderful cleanser and anti-inflammatory beverage, carrot juice is rich in vitamins and minerals— for example, vitamin A, which is noted for its benefit in healing infection.
- Give plenty of spring water to drink.
- Apply a compress as hot as tolerable to the styes and the surrounding area. The heat will help bring them to the surface and drain. Sometimes styes resolve simply by reducing in size. Repeat at least twice, preferably four times, a day. Herbal compresses are ideal, but hot-water compresses will certainly suffice.

Herbal Recommendations

- To make a compress from herbs, you merely use hot tea instead of hot water. An excellent choice for reducing inflammation and infection is chamomile tea (1 tablespoon herb to 1 cup hot water) to which 1/4 teaspoon goldenseal powder has been added. Steep for twenty minutes, strain well, and apply. This solution can be reheated over the course of the day and then discarded. Prepare fresh daily. Other herbs that can be used as compresses include calendula, eyebright, rosemary, and chickweed, alone or in combination.
- Between compresses you can rinse the eyes periodically with cool water to reduce itching.
- Internally give 20 drops of echinacea and 250 to 500 milligrams vitamin C a few times each day. Your child also can drink anti-inflammatory herbal infusions made with burdock root, chickweed, red clover blossoms, or plantain leaf.

❖ Sunburn ❖

There is a lot of controversy over how much exposure to the sun is safe, and there are hundreds of products available to protect us from the sun's "harmful rays." The incidence of skin cancers is apparently rising, and with the depletion of the ozone layer, some scientists have claimed that this trend is likely to continue. Sunburn is a result of overexposure to the sun, but whether it is the sole cause of skin cancer is unknown. The synthetic chemicals in our diets that we sweat out through the skin, the synthetic creams and lotions that we slather on ourselves, and the many airborne chemicals that leave residue on the skin may be factors as well. But it is clear that sitting in the sun, baking in a coating of suntan lotion containing who knows what, no matter how much sunscreen it contains, is not without health risk. Nevertheless, sunshine is essential to health in many ways. Emotionally, we feel uplifted and energized when we enjoy the sun's warmth and light. Physically, exposure to the sun provides us with the ability to sythesize vitamin D, a necessary component for calcium absorption and thus bone growth and development. We probably don't even know all the factors essential for health that depend upon our exposure to sunlight.

Obviously, then, some exposure to sunlight is necessary, although we need to protect ourselves and our children from the harmful effects of overexposure. To reduce the risk of sunburn (and avoid the who-knows-whats on your children's skin) use only 100 percent natural sunscreens (read labels!), and teach your children to recognize when they've had enough sun, particularly at the beach. You will have to look out for the younger ones and remind older kids. Children with sensitive skin should wear a T-shirt in the water, especially the first few times they swim in the season. A wide-brimmed sun hat will help protect the face, shoulders, and upper back, the most likely areas to become burned.

Cocoa butter is an excellent skin softener and moisturizer after exposure. Coconut oil can be used the same way. Moisturizing the skin whether or not there has been any burning is a good way to replenish lost nutrients and protect the skin from becoming dry or itchy. In the long run, this practice can help the skin stay healthy.

WHEN TO SEEK MEDICAL CARE

High fever in conjunction with overexposure to the sun can mean heatstroke. This is a medical emergency. Immediately cool the child with very cold water while transporting him or her to the nearest hospital. Any serious burns, especially in very young children and babies, should be given careful attention.

HERBAL RECOMMENDATIONS

- Cool the skin with water before treating; then apply aloe vera gel, calendula cream or oil, or St. John's wort oil. Aloe vera gel is a sunburn treatment par excellence. You can purchase it in a bottle and carry it along with you, or you can keep an aloe plant at home, breaking off leaves as you need them, slicing them open and scraping out the pulp inside to rub on the burn. This can be repeated as often as necessary.

- Give your child extra fluids to drink, and, if a low fever develops, treat accordingly with cooling herbs such as peppermint, lemon balm, catnip, or other herbs discussed in "Fevers."

Relaxing teas can help your child get comfortable and rest. If necessary, refer to "Burns."

❖ TICKS ❖

Ticks can be found in most areas of the United States. Most often, you discover a tick bite by finding the insect itself burrowing into the skin. These readily visible, common ticks, however, do not carry Lyme disease, the most prominent tick-borne disease, which is contracted through deer ticks. These extremely small insects often go unnoticed. If you notice any red patches on the skin that resemble a "bull's eye," especially after being in an area known to have deer ticks, seek medical evaluation. Within a couple of days the red patch may become a lesion or the child may exhibit flulike symptoms—further evidence of Lyme disease.

Diagnosis of the disease is made by a blood test, the results of which will be positive several weeks after the tick bite. Treatment is based on the severity of the illness. Some people develop only a mild case with the initial symptoms, while others may have more serious problems like chronic fatigue and arthritis. Depending upon the seriousness of the case, you may choose to use natural remedies to allay the symptoms and strengthen immunity or a combination of natural remedies and pharmaceutical drugs. It is a good idea to be know if Lyme disease is prevalent in your area or in areas where you may travel; early diagnosis and treatment may reduce the severity of the problem.

If you find any type of tick on your child's body, first smother it in oil or rubbing alcohol. Then grasp it by the head with tweezers, or, if necessary, your fingers, and pull it out with a twisting motion. If no oil or alcohol is available, remove it anyway. To avoid infection, be sure to get all of the insect out. If you suspect that it is a disease-carrying tick, save it for further identification. If not, dispose of it by flushing it down the toilet or crushing it.

After removing the tick, wash the area well with an antiseptic solution such as apple cider vinegar or a tincture of calendula, echinacea, or rosemary. Echinacea, garlic, thyme, or cleavers may be given internally as well. Observe for signs of infection and attend to accordingly.

❖ Urinary-Tract Infections ❖

Urinary-tract infections (UTIs) affect the bladder, urethra (pee-hole), and kidneys. Most commonly they start out as simple bladder infections that, if treated promptly, do not progress to a more serious kidney infection. Signs of a UTI can include some or all of these symptoms: frequent urination, often with a burning sensation; need to pee often with little coming out; low-backache or bellyache (probably the first thing you'll notice is that your child is going to the bathroom a lot more often than usual); vaginal bleeding; and, occasionally, fever, chills, and malaise.

Little girls are more susceptible than boys to UTIs because bacteria from the rectum are more likely to enter the urethra. Drafts from wearing skirts with inadequately warm undergarments also can cause UTIs. To prevent them, have your daughter wear warm pants or tights in winter so she doesn't develop a chill, and teach her to wipe from front to back after using the toilet. The latter habit prevents the spread of bacteria from the anus to the urethra, bladder, and vaginal canal. Also, explain that she should pee as soon as she can rather than holding it. Other causes of UTIs are bubble baths, scented toilet paper, and synthetic fibers in tights and underwear, all of which instigate infection by causing local irritation.

A vaginal yeast infection that is causing itching can irritate the urethra and lead to a UTI. If you suspect a yeast infection, see "Thrush" in Chapter 7.

WHEN TO SEEK MEDICAL CARE

Kidney infections can be quite serious. If your child has shown symptoms of a UTI and seems very sick or in a lot of pain, seek an experienced caregiver immediately. Likewise, if symptoms worsen or show no improvement despite home treatment, seek further care.

DIETARY AND HERBAL RECOMMENDATIONS

Mild bladder infections can be dealt with at home. The real key is in early treatment. The following remedies, if used in combination as a routine, should noticeably improve the child's health within twenty-four hours, and the infection should totally clear up within a week. Treat until all symptoms are gone, then for an additional two days.

- Give copious quantities of water and nettles infusion throughout the day. Fresh carrot juice is also good. Up to a half gallon of liquid a day is ideal. Water helps flush the infection from the system by diluting the urine and also by washing the bladder as more urine is produced and passed. This dilution of the urine also serves to reduce any burning. Nettles strengthens the kidneys and keeps infection from ascending toward them.

- Unsweetened cranberry juice should be drunk daily, up to six glasses a day (include as part of the day's overall fluid intake). Cranberry juice changes the pH of the urine, making it unfavorable to the bacteria, and may actually contain antibiotic properties. If your child finds the juice unbearably sour, dilute it with an equal quantity of unsweetened natural apple juice.
- Give 500 milligrams of vitamin C and 10 to 30 drops of echinacea tincture four times a day.
- Both uva ursi and yarrow are known to be urinary antiseptics and are strengthening to the urinary tract. Either alone or combined with each other, they are specifically used to treat urinary-tract infections. To prepare, steep 1 ounce of either or a combination of equal parts of both in a quart of boiling water for up to two hours. Strain and give 1/8 to 1/2 cup of the infusion (the older and heavier the child, the more you should give) four times daily.
- If your child is experiencing a lot of burning when he or she pees, add a couple of tablespoons of either marshmallow or comfrey root to the above infusion. These mucilaginous herbs reduce inflammation and discomfort.
- The diet should be simple and free of sweeteners and dessert-type foods as these tend to aggravate UTIs. Whole grains, high-quality protein foods (legumes, nuts, seeds, and fish, for example), and lots of fresh vegetables are ideal.

If your child suffers from frequent urinary-tract infections, try the above suggestions for the immediate flare-up. Make appropriate changes to eliminate the causes of the infection as discussed at the beginning of this section. Don't dismiss emotional issues that may be at the heart of the matter. (The expression *pissed off* may give you a clue: Is there something angering your child? Language coincidences may be more relevant than we suspect.)

Herbs such as chickweed, burdock root, dandelion leaf and root, and cleavers can help reduce heat in the body and can be given regularly as infusions, up to a cup a day for a few weeks, to prevent recurrence. Tinctures of these herbs can also be used with good results.

❖ Vaginal Itching ❖

Girls may occasionally experience itching in the vaginal canal or vulva. Henceforth, I will also use the word *yoni* for these terms, based on the sacred Sanskrit word for *genitalia*, as opposed to the word *vagina*, which means "sheath." We need not always see our bodies in relationship to men or as merely available to serve them, as implied by the idea that our genitalia are intended to hold a sword!

Much like urinary-tract infections, vaginal itching can be caused by the chemicals in bubble baths, soaps, detergents, and perfumed toilet paper; tight-fitting or synthetic underwear, tights, or pants; a wet bathing suit; transference of bacteria from the rectum to the yoni; inadequate bathing; and contact with unclean hands. Teaching girls to love and respect their bodies from an early age is an important gift that we can give them to help ensure their health. So many problems in our society, such as anorexia/bulimia, drug abuse, and sexual diseases, stem from disrespect of our bodies. Help your daughter to be comfortable with and knowledgeable about her whole self, including her genitals. This instruction will serve her for her lifetime!

A yeast infection can cause persistent itching. If your child has a slightly curdy or cheesy discharge that smells faintly like yeasted bread, you can surmise that yeast is the source of the problem. Any of the culprits mentioned above can lead to a yeast infection. So can recent use of antibiotics or a diet high in sweets and simple carbohydrates (like white-flour products; whole grains are complex carbohydrates).

Another cause of severe itching and even pain is vaginal pinworms. These small intestinal parasites can migrate to the yoni and get inside causing discomfort ranging from mild to extreme. If you suspect this condition, see "Intestinal Parasites." To eliminate the discomfort and get the worms to leave the genital area, have your daughter soak in a bath to which has been added 1 cup of Epsom salts. She should do this daily until the problem clears up.

General Recommendations

- Discontinue use of any product mentioned above (bubble bath, scented toilet paper, and so forth) that are heavily perfumed and can lead to a reaction. Even many natural bubble-bath products are strong and cause reactions in little girls. Aloe vera–based products are often mild and nonirritating.
- Replace nylon panties and tights with breathable cotton. Nylon traps moisture, encouraging the growth of yeast and bacteria.
- Teach your daughter to wash herself thoroughly, especially in warm

weather. Soap may irritate her bottom; plain water is adequate. Always wash your children gently; you are sending them a message of how they deserve to be treated. As soon as she's old enough, let her wash herself.

- Silly as it may seem, a lot of women, let alone girls, don't know that they should wipe from front to back when they use the bathroom. Bacteria that live in the rectum can cause a lot of irritation and even infection when they enter the yoni, so teach your child proper toilet hygiene.

DIETARY RECOMMENDATIONS

- Reduce sugar in all forms until the discomfort clears up, allowing only occasional fruit. Eliminate juices, pastries, and candies. Allow only one or two pieces of fresh fruit in season per day. Temporarily avoid yeasted products as well: they tend to aggravate yeast-related genital itching.
- Give your daughter plenty of water to drink.

HERBAL RECOMMENDATIONS

- For irritation that seems related to yeast infection, refer to "Thrush" in Chapter 7. Also, let your daughter wash her yoni with unsweetened natural yogurt with active cultures. Let it come to room temperature first, or the coldness will be startling. She can apply it with a washcloth and then rinse it off in a bath. Yogurt is soothing to inflammation and restores the natural acid-alkaline balance and natural flora of the area.
- For general itching herbal baths are soothing. Apply healing salve, calendula oil, slippery elm bark powder (sprinkled onto the area), aloe vera gel, or compresses made with chamomile, calendula, or chickweed for relief of discomfort and irritation.

❖ VOMITING ❖

Vomiting is very direct way for the body to clean out the stomach, be it from too much food, contaminated food, or a stomach virus, and is usually not a cause for worry. It also occurs as a reaction to overstimulation.

DEHYDRATION DANGER

In an otherwise-healthy child the greatest risk associated with persistent vomiting is dehydration, which can be dangerous and must be treated quickly. Your main concern should be to give your child plenty of fluids to prevent it from occurring. Signs of dehydration include a dry tongue and oral mucous membranes (such as the insides of the cheeks), little or no urine output, dark urine, sudden weight loss, sunken and dry eyes, sunken fontanel (the soft spot on a baby's head), loss of skin elasticity, and, in serious cases, fast pulse and fever.

WHEN TO SEEK MEDICAL CARE

Vomiting associated with a head injury or other symptoms like severe headache and stiff neck or severe abdominal pain can be a sign of very serious illness. Seek immediate medical care.

Babies who are rejecting all fluids and won't breast-feed need careful attention because they can become dehydrated quickly. Newborns who vomit repeatedly may have a congenital problem and should be seen immediately by a pediatrician.

Be aware that frequent vomiting in teenagers, both girls and boys, may be deliberate and is a sign of bulimia, a serious eating disorder. If you suspect this condition, find supportive counseling for you and your child so you can work together to address the heart of the problem. Eating disorders are life threatening!

GENERAL RECOMMENDATIONS

- Since drinking large amounts of fluids at once often aggravates the stomach and is thrown up, give frequent, small doses of fluids. Giving 1 or 2 tablespoons of liquid every ten minutes should be sufficient. Liquids can include water at room temperature, slightly salty broth, herbal teas as follows, an electrolyte replacement drink such as "Recharge," or "Third Wind," or the homemade recipe described below. The most important thing is for your child to drink, so whatever beverages will stay down are appropriate.

  You can prepare a homemade electrolyte replacement drink by mixing 8 ounces of water (warm or at room temperature); 1/4 teaspoon baking soda; 1 pinch of salt; and honey, sugar, or maple syrup to taste (at least 2 teaspoons). Never give honey to children under a year old. You can administer the drink by tablespoon often or by the quarter or half cup every half hour or so.

- Keep your child feeling as fresh and clean as possible, and keep the environment tranquil. A mister bottle filled with water and a few drops of essential oil such as lavender, rose, lemon, or eucalyptus can freshen up the room, which is likely to take on a stale smell from the vomiting.

- One of the most remarkable treatments for persistent vomiting is the hot salt pack. The purpose is to send heat to the hollow organ of the stomach and to reduce cramping and spasms. Applied directly over the stomach (not over the whole belly), it can arrest vomiting after just a few treatments.

  To prepare a salt pack, heat 1 cup of natural sea salt in a skillet for three to five minutes or until very hot. Pour the salt into a sack (like an old pillow case) and then fold the sack until you have a pack of salt about the area of your child's stomach. Wrap the sack in a thin towel to prevent it from burning the skin (salt gets incredibly hot) and apply. If your child says it is too hot, wrap the sack in a slightly thicker towel. You want the treatment to be as warm as tolerable but not burning.

  Keep it on until comfort is achieved, and reapply after a rest of at least thirty minutes, by reheating the same salt and repeating the procedure.

HERBAL RECOMMENDATIONS

- Herbs helpful for vomiting either relax the child and the stomach, thus preventing stomach spasms and nausea, or they warm the stomach, which serves the same function. Prepare teas of any of these herbs alone or in combination: ginger root, cinnamon, chamomile, catnip, lemon balm. The addition of a small amount of spearmint or peppermint can also reduce nausea. In the case of dysentery or a stomach virus, add antimicrobial herbs such as echinacea or small amounts of goldenseal. Tincture can be used, 10 to 30 drops of echinacea, and/or 5 to 15 drops of goldenseal, every two to four hours depending upon the severity of the illness.
- Ume-Sho-Kudzu is very easy to digest, is delicious, and helps reduce vomiting. To prepare, dissolve a large teaspoon of kudzu powder in 2 tablespoons cold water. Crush the pulp of one umeboshi plum (or 1/2 teaspoon of umeboshi plum paste). Add these ingredients to 1 1/2 to 2 cups cold water and bring to a boil, stirring constantly. Add 1/2 teaspoon of freshly grated ginger juice or ginger powder. Add 1 to 3 teaspoons of tamari soy sauce and boil a minute longer. Serve when cool enough to drink but still quite warm.

❖ WHOOPING COUGH (PERTUSSIS) ❖

Whooping cough, or pertussis (so named for the bacteria, *Bortadella pertussis*, that triggers it), is one of the illnesses children are routinely vaccinated against. It is the *P* in DPT, the diptheria, pertussis, and teta-nus vaccine. Because of the vaccine's relatively high incidence of tragic reactions, including permanent brain damage and death, many parents are choosing not to give this immunization. In addition, the vaccine is not even 100 percent effective. Consequently, whooping cough may be more prevalent than expected.

Whooping cough begins as a typical cold with a cough and is most commonly seen in the late winter and early spring. Over a period of time, for some a few days but for most a week or two, the cough becomes progressively worse until the child has full-blown coughing fits (known as "paroxysmal coughing"). During these episodes the child may seem unable to catch his breath, his face may become red or purple from the sheer effort, and often the bout will end with the child vomiting. Mucus may or may not be brought up with the cough. The coughing fits may occur infrequently or can recur many times throughout the day and night. It is during these fits that the characteristic "whooping" sound is heard. This second stage of whooping cough can persist for weeks or months, during which time the cough gradually abates. A mild cough may linger for quite some time. The child may be quite exhausted, increasing his or her susceptibility to other infections. In Chinese medicine, one of the names for whooping cough is "the hundred days cough."

Not all children who are exposed to pertussis will become as sick as just described. The strength of the child's constitution as well as current health status and age are significant factors. The younger the child, the greater the likelihood of complications, especially when the child is un-der three years.

Whooping cough is spread primarily through water droplets from coughing and sneezing. If your child has been exposed to someone who has this illness (and don't discount adults—they can get it, too), begin preventive treatment. If you catch it at the onset, you can lessen the severity of the second stage if it develops at all. This is a good time to build the immune system and to use antimicrobial herbs.

Once the whoop sets in, antibiotics can do nothing about the pertussis itself because the cough is then caused by chemical irritants released as the bacteria break down, not by the bacteria themselves. They can, however, prevent secondary infections like pneumonia from developing. Older chil-dren and adults can usually manage well without antibiotics, but they may be perfectly appropriate for small children and those who are already frail.

Interestingly, another term from traditional Chinese medicine used to describe whooping cough is "the cough of enlightenment." It is said that the illness puts the child through a spiritual trial from which he or she emerges more peaceful and patient. Parents I know whose children have had whooping cough confirm this. While none would wish it on another, perhaps whooping cough and other illnesses serve a greater psychic and spiritual purpose than we are aware of.

Nevertheless, this illness is frightening and tiring for both child and parents, who have to stay close at all times to maintain the child's general well-being while trying to reduce the frequency and severity of the cough. Though whopping cough is rarely dangerous, it is at best exhausting to children, at worst it can lead to choking or hernia in very young kids. Of course, if your child seems seriously compromised at any time during the illness, seek immediate medical care.

DIETARY RECOMMENDATIONS

- At the onset of any cold it is best to simplify the diet. Getting down to basics—whole grains and steamed vegetables, warm beverages, soups, and porridges—are always a good bet. Small amounts of legumes or light meat such as poultry and fish can supply a good nutrient boost that raises the body's ability to heal infection. As whooping cough can be a prolonged and weakening illness, these protein foods are important for restoring vitality and strength.
- During the early stages of the illness, don't force the child to eat much if he is not hungry; this is a perfectly natural response, and the appetite usually returns of its own accord. If the appetite loss persists, give a few drops of dandelion root or agrimony tincture to stimulate digestive activity. Give 10 to 20 drops in warm water a few times a day until the appetite returns.
- Fluids are essential at all times. At no time should a sick child go without fluids. Warm beverages are preferable; choose any of the general-purpose teas and broths mentioned for general health in this book.

HERBAL RECOMMENDATIONS

- To reduce the likelihood of a full-blown case of whooping cough, begin herbal care as soon as possible after a suspected or known exposure. Use an herbal approach combining a few different remedies to address your child's needs as he enters the various stages of the illness.
- Since homeopathic remedies are simple to give and most kids love to suck on the sweet pellets, including them as a part of your

health plan is easy. Homeopathic aconite 6x or 30x and homeopathic belladonna 6x or 30x are indicated for illnesses that have sudden onset after exposure to wind, as may often be the case with pertussis, and may be given at the onset of the cold symptoms. Homeopathic droesera (sundew) 30x and the preparation called pertussin 30x are specifically indicated during whooping cough. The general dosage is 3 to 5 pellets up to every two hours in difficult cases, or four times a day until relief is found. If no response is noticed after a few doses, a different homeopathic remedy may better suit your child. Specifics about homeopathy are beyond the scope of this book, so you will need to consult reference books and local practitioners.

- Use of garlic, echinacea, and vitamin C can reduce the severity of most infectious diseases and the likelihood of secondary complications. Whooping cough is no exception. Give echinacea in tincture form (glycerin macerate, which contains no alcohol and is sweet tasting, may also be used with kids), 20 to 35 drops every few hours during the acute phases of the illness and 10 to 20 drops three times a day during the recovery period. Give 250 to 500 milligrams vitamin C four times a day. Foods high in this vitamin also should be included in the diet. Examples are dark leafy greens and broccoli, cantaloupe, strawberries, rosehips, alfalfa sprouts, and, of course, citrus and tomatoes (these last two should be used in small quantities). Raw garlic can be given in several ways: chopped and mixed with a teaspoon with honey, in garlic lemonade (see recipes in "Colds and Flu"), or in garlic perles available at natural-food stores. Give as much garlic as possible as long as it is not causing digestive upset. If the child can take a few cloves a day, that is ideal.

- The following two preparations can be used alone, interchangeably, or in combination. One is an infusion, the other a syrup.

"Whoop-ease" Tea: Mix 1/2 ounce each of thyme, red clover blossoms, and marshmallow root and place in a quart-size Mason jar. Cover with 1 quart boiling water and cap the jar. Steep for two hours, strain, and add 1/4 cup honey. Give in doses of 1 tablespoon to 1/2 cup at a time, up to 1 quart daily.

Thyme is an antimicrobial herb particularly beneficial for lung infections. Its volatile oils, which give it its characteristic aroma, ease and relax the respiratory passages and make the child more comfortable. It aids expectoration, eases sore throats, and stimulates sluggish digestion. Red clover blossoms are gently expectorant and antispasmodic. They are also in the category of herbs that purify the blood. Marshmallow root aids expectoration as it reduces inflammation and irritation of the bronchi and lungs as well as the throat.

Cough and lung syrup: Mix the following dried herbs and store in a jar or bag away from heat and light: 1/4 ounce each of colts-foot (not safe for pregnant women!), burdock root, mullein leaf, marshmallow root, licorice root, thyme, and anise seed; 1/8 ounce of wild cherry bark. Add 1/16 ounce each of slippery elm bark and lobelia. Put 1 ounce of this mix into a quart-size jar. Fill the jar with boiling water and steep for four to six hours. Strain the liquid into a measuring cup and discard or compost the herb material. After noting how much liquid you have, pour it into a small pan and simmer uncovered until the liquid is reduced to 1 cup. To this add 1/4 cup honey and stir well. Let cool to room temperature; then store in the refrigerator. Give up to 2 tablespoons every two hours.

The herbs in this syrup relax and soothe a child's lungs when he or she has been suffering from frequent and intense coughing. They quiet the cough while moistening the throat and reducing inflammation. Because they are sweet and concentrated, syrups allow you to give a larger amount of a formula in a smaller dose, ideal for small children or remedies using strong-tasting herbs. In the case of whooping cough, you may want to give a small amount of syrup frequently to keep the coughing to a minimum. You can prepare Whoop-Ease Tea as a syrup as described above.

- Mustard plasters are an exceptional remedy for children over two years old who have a lot of lung congestion and are troubled by frequent coughing spells. I have seen them used with bronchitis and whooping cough, in the latter case bringing sleep and comfort to a nine-year-old boy (and his parents!) for a five-hour stretch, whereas on previous nights he was waking every thirty minutes with severe coughing. See "Herbal Preparations" in Chapter 4 for instructions. Mustard is very irritating to the skin, so be careful to follow all precautions.

- Add thyme in infusion or a few drops of the oil to hot bathwater. This is an excellent remedy especially for babies and young children because you don't have to get them to take anything, and little ones usually love to linger in the tub. You can give your child a bath a couple times a day if needed.

- Of course, teas such as chamomile and lemon balm as well as other calming teas can be used to comfort and relax the child.

During the course of whooping cough there may be periods of time each day when your child needs you urgently. He or she needs a lot of closeness and reassurance during coughing spells but may seem perfectly fine between them. Keeping your child at home for the first few weeks of illness, even if only one coughing bout occurs each day, is extremely important. Not only is it a highly contagious illness, but it is also demanding of the child in both body and spirit. The child should be kept restful, and until resistance to further illness is strong, staying home is wisest. Fresh air and going outside for short periods each day are great provided the air is warm and the day is not windy.

If your child is quite ill and you are the primary-care provider, arrange for some time on a regular basis when you can refresh and restore yourself so you don't become thoroughly exhausted. If your child wakes frequently at night, you can take naps together during the day. Sleeping in the same room, even snuggled together at night, can be reassuring to your child and enables you to rest easier because you are nearby and know your child is okay. This may make nighttime go more smoothly.

After the worst of the illness has passed, provide your child with 1–2 cups a day of the following respiratory tonic to rebuild the strength of the lungs and prevent subsequent illnesses. This recipe was created by Rosemary Gladstar Slick and was originally published in her booklet, "Herbs for Children."

Respiratory Tonic: Mix together and store in a jar 1/2 ounce each of red clover blossoms, comfrey leaves, mullein leaves, coltsfoot (UNSAFE FOR USE DURING PREGNANCY), and calendula flowers, and 1/4 ounce each of lemon grass, rosehips, and fennel seeds. Steep one handful of the mix per quart of boiling water for fifteen to twenty minutes. Strain, sweeten if desired, and drink. This mix makes a refreshing summer iced tea as well as a hot medicinal drink.

Note: Frequently a child who has just recovered from whooping cough will "whoop" the next time he or she has a cold. This is normal and is not a relapse of the pertussis; whooping cough rarely occurs more than once.

Appendix I

❖

Common and Latin Names for Herbs

Many plants may have the same common name, and any given plant may have a number of common names. A plant's Latin name (also known as the "botanical" or "horticultural" name) is its internationally recognized name. When purchasing herbs, check their Latin names to ensure that you are using the correct plant in your herbal preparations.

Common Name	Latin Name
Agrimony	*Agrimonia eupatoria*
Alfalfa	*Medicago sativa*
Angelica	*Angelica archangelica*
Anise	*Pimpinella anisum*
Arnica	*Arnica montana*
Astragalus	*Astragalus mongolicus*
Bayberry bark	*Myrica cerifera*
Blackberry	*Rubus idaeus*
Black currant	*Ribes nigrum*
Black walnut	*Juglans nigra*
Blessed thistle	*Cnicus benedictus*
Blue cohosh	*Caulophyllum thalictroides*
Borage	*Borago officinalis*
Burdock	*Arctium lappa*
Calendula	*Calendula officinalis*
Catnip	*Nepeta cataria*
Chamomile	*Anthemis nobilis; Matriarca chamomilla*
Chaparral	*Larrea divaricata*
Chickweed	*Stellaria media*
Chrysanthemum	*Chrysanthemum morifolium*
Cleavers	*Galium aparine*
Cinnamon	*Cinnamomum zeylanicum*
Codonopsis	*Codonopsis pilosula*
Coltsfoot	*Tussilago farfara*
Comfrey	*Symphytum officinale*
Cramp Bark	*Viburnum opulus*
Dandelion	*Taraxacum officinale*
Echinacea	*Echinacea angustifolia*
Elder	*Sambucus nigra*
Elecampane	*Inula helenium*

Common Name	Latin Name
Ephedra	*Ephedra sinica*
Eyebright	*Euphrasia officinalis*
False unicorn	*Chamaelirium luteum*
Fennel	*Foeniculum vulgare*
Fenugreek	*Trigonella foenum-graecum*
Flax seed	*Linum usitatissimum*
Garlic	*Allium sativum*
Ginger	*Zingiber officinale*
Goldenseal	*Hydrastis canadensis*
Hawthorn	*Crataegus oxyacantha*
Hops	*Humulus lupulus*
Horehound	*Marrubium vulgare*
Horsetail	*Equisetum arvense*
Irish moss	*Chondrus crispus*
Jewel weed	*Impatiens aurea*
Kudzu	*Pueraria lobata et thunbergiana*
Lady's slipper	*Cypripedium pubescens*
Lavender	*Lavandula officinalis*
Lemon balm	*Melissa officinalis*
Lemon grass	*Cymbopogon citratus*
Licorice	*Glycyrrhiza glabra*
Lime blossom	*Tilia europaea*
Lobelia	*Lobelia inflata*
Marshmallow	*Althaea officinalis*
Motherwort	*Leonorus cardiaca*
Mullein	*Verbascum thapsus*
Myrrh	*Commiphora myrrha*
Nasturtium	*Trapaeolum majus*
Nettles	*Urtica dioica*
Oatstraw	*Avena sativa*
Parsley	*Petroselinum crispum*
Peppermint	*Mentha piperita*
Plantain	*Plantago major, P. lanceolata*
Red clover	*Trifolium pratense*
Red raspberry	*Rubus idaeus*
Rose	*Rosa canina*
Rosemary	*Rosmarinus officinalis*
Rue	*Ruta graveolens*
Sage	*Salvia officinalis*
Sarsaparilla	*Smilax officinalis*
Sassafras	*Sassafras officinale*
Shepherd's purse	*Capsella bursa-pastoris*
Skullcap	*Scutellaria laterifolia*
Slippery elm	*Ulmus fulva*
Squawvine	*Mitchella repens*
St. John's wort	*Hypericum perforatum*

Common Name	Latin Name
Strawberry	*Fragaria* species
Thyme	*Thymus vulgaris*
Uva ursi	*Arctostaphylos uva ursi*
Valerian	*Valeriana officinalis*
Vervain	*Verbena officinalis*
Violet	*Viola* species
White oak	*Quercus alba*
Wild cherry	*Prunus serotina*
Wild yam	*Doscorea villosa*
Witch hazel	*Hamamelis virginiana*
Wormwood	*Artemisia absinthium*
Yarrow	*Achillea millefolium*
Yellow dock	*Rumex crispus*

Appendix II

❖

Herbal First-Aid Kit

Herbs can relieve minor injuries like cuts, first-degree burns, and insect bites and sometimes can assist with more serious conditions. The kit described below covers a wide range of situations; in fact, it was designed for use by our family on camping trips to provide first-aid for minor injuries and immediate care when an emergency room is not just up the road. It also supplements our home herbal medicine chest.

This kit does *not* replace conventional medical care, the best option for emergencies. *Always seek emergency medical care as soon as possible when a situation is beyond your scope or knowledge and if a person is in danger!*

Training in basic first-aid procedures, available through the American Red Cross, is highly recommended. Also from the Red Cross you can obtain a basic first-aid manual, which you should read and keep in your kit. Contact your local chapter for information.

A standard metal tool or tackle box is a convenient and safe way to store and transport your first-aid supplies. Herb powders, ointments, and tinctures can be kept in 1-ounce bottles or tins available from suppliers of herbal products (see "Resources"). Most of the herbs listed keep for a year; tinctures keep longer—up to four years—providing they are stored in a cool spot. Always check the contents and freshness of your kit before a journey. It won't do you any good if it's half-empty or spoiled.

❖ HERBAL SUPPLIES ❖

Tinctures (1 ounce of each)

echinacea

goldenseal

calendula

dandelion

skullcap

bayberry bark–shepherd's purse

cayenne pepper

ipecac syrup

Bach Rescue Remedy (Bach Flower essence)

plaintain

chickweed–burdock root–plantain

Antispasmodic Tincture (Herb Pharm)

Children's Compound (Herb Pharm)

Calm Child Formula (Planetary Formulas)

Ointments and Oils (1 ounce of each)

calendula oil
arnica oil
garlic-mullein oil
St. John's wort oil
plantain oil

aloe vera gel
Peppermint oil (1/2 ounce)
herbal salve
Tiger Balm

Herbal Powders (about 2 tablespoons each)

slippery elm
ginger root
comfrey root

green clay
goldenseal-echinacea-chaparral

Miscellaneous

"00" capsules (20)
insect repellent
lip balm
activated charcoal
   tablets (50)
raw honey (a few tablespoons)

vitamin C, 500-milligram chewables (50)
vitamin E, 400 IU capsules (20)
homeopathic remedies: arnica, aconite,
   rhus tox. (all 30x)
umeboshi plum paste (a small amount)

❖ NONHERBAL SUPPLIES ❖

bandages (assorted sizes)
elastic roll bandage
sterile gauze pads ("4 | 4")
adhesive tape
cotton balls
cotton swabs
oral thermometer
small, sharp scissors
latex gloves

butterfly bandages
finger splint
tweezers
matches
hydrogen peroxide
snake-bite kit (optional)
epinephrine kit (for bee allergy)
hot and cold compresses
first-aid manual

Resources

❖ BULK HERBS, HERBAL PRODUCTS, BOOKS, AND SUPPLIES ❖

Catalogs are available from all of these companies.

Avena Botanicals
219 Mill Street
Rockport, ME 04856
Bulk herbs, tinctures, books, classes, and more.

Cascade Health Care Products
141 Commercial Street, NE
Salem, OR 97301
800-443-9942
Complete line of health products for pregnant women and midwives as well as many for babies and kids; good source of moxibustion supplies and books on many areas of pregnancy and child health.

Frontier Cooperative Herbs
P.O. Box 299
Norway, IA 52318
800-669-3275
Bulk herbs and health and beauty products at wholesale prices.

Herb Pharm
P.O. Box 116
Williams, OR 97544
800-348-4372
The highest-quality tinctures available.

Mountain Rose Herbs
P.O. Box 2000
Redway, CA 95560
800-879-3337
Beautiful catalog of bulk herbs, jars and tins, books, and premade formulas.

Mountain Spirit
P.O. Box 368
Port Townsend, WA 98368
360-385-4491
Herbs, spiritual tools, and books.

Penn Herbs
603 North Second Street
Philadelphia, PA 19123
800-523-9971
A good source for hard-to-find powdered herbs.

Wish Garden Herbs
1308 Kilkenny Road
Boulder, CO 80303
303-665-9508
A home business that supplies high-quality and hard-to-find herb tinctures, especially for moms and midwives.

❖ Chinese Herbs, Books, and Supplies ❖

Some of the companies listed above also sell these products, but the following carry a wide range of Chinese herbal and medical supplies.

Brion Herbs
9250 Jeronimo Road
Irvine, CA 92718
714-587-1238 or 800-283-5191
This is the distributor of Sun Ten Herbal Formulas, an excellent Chinese herbal product that comes freeze-dried and is easy to give to kids.

The Herb Shoppe
4372 Chris Greene Lake Road
Charlottesville, VA 22901
804-973-1700
Herbalist Paul Olko specializes in custom blends of both Western and Chinese herbs and keeps a large variety of herbs in stock.

Redwing/Meridian
44 Linden Street
Brookline, MA 02146
800-873-3946 or 800-356-6003
A great source of lay and technical books on traditional Chinese medicine as well as herbs.

❖ Miscellaneous ❖

Bushy Mountain Bee Company
800-BEESWAX
The best supplier with the lowest prices! A must for salve making.

Doulas of North America
1100 Twenty-third Avenue East
Seattle, WA 98112
This organization offers training in the postpartum support of new mothers.

Hearthsong
156 North Main Street
Sebastopol, CA 95472
800-325-2502
Beautiful naturally made toys, crafts, and books for children and teens. Expensive but high quality.

Homeopathic Educational Services
2124 Kittredge Street
Berkeley, CA 94704
207-594-0694
An excellent catalog filled with information about kid's health.

La Leche League International
800-LA LECHE
Complete breast-feeding and parenting information for mothers whether they stay at home or work at outside jobs.

Maine Seaweed Company
P.O. Box 57
Steuben, ME 04680
207-546-2875
Excellent sea vegetables harvested with complete respect for the health of the ocean.

John Holt's Book and Music Store
2269 Massacusetts Avenue
Cambridge, MA 02140
617-843-3100
Great books and ideas for homeschoolers. A magazine is available, too.

❖ HOME-STUDY OPPORTUNITIES IN HEALTH AND HERBALISM ❖

Michael Tierra, C.A., and Lesley Tierra, C.A.
East West Herb Course
P.O. Box 712
Santa Cruz, CA 95061

This study course enables the student to develop working knowledge in the fundamentals of health and herbalism. A more extensive master course gives students complete training in Chinese and Western herbalism.

Hygieia College
P.O. Box 398
Monroe, UT 84754
801-527-3738
Jeannine Parvati Baker is the founder of this program, which is "a college in the original meaning, that is in a grove of trees, which is a state of mind. . . ." Lessons in womancraft, herbalism, and midwifery are available via mail. Baker is the author of a number of books, including *Hygieia: A Woman's Herbal* and *Prenatal Yoga and Natural Birth,* and a coauthor of *Conscious Conception.*

Sage Mountain
P.O. Box 420-M
East Barre, VT 05649
802-479-9825
Rosemary Gladstar Slick, founder of the California School of Herbal Studies, is a pioneer woman herbalist and author of numerous booklets on herbs for women, men, and children. She offers a correspondence course in herbal studies, for which you can get information by contacting the above address.

Susun S. Weed
Wise Woman Center
P.O. Box 64-M
Woodstock, NY 12498
914-246-8081
Susun Weed, author of *Healing Wise, Wise Woman Herbal for the Childbearing Year,* and *Menopausal Years,* offers workshops and apprenticeships at her home and travels internationally on speaking engagements.

Dr. George Wootan
P.O. Box 270
Hurley, NY 12443
800-635-2126
Dr. Wootan teaches an excellent weekend course called "Pediatrics for Parents," which you can sponsor where you live. I highly recommend it. Dr. Wootan is the author of *Take Charge of Your Child's Health,* which can be purchased directly through him at the address listed above and is a must for your library.

Further Reading

The books listed below enable you to expand your knowledge and awareness of natural health care and deepen your understanding of the political and historical roots of health and healing.

❖ PARENTING AND CHILDREN'S HEALTH ❖

See "General Herbalism" for children's herbals.

Armstrong, Liz, and Adrienne Scott. *Whitewash.* Toronto: HarperCollins, 1992.

Baldwin, Rahima. *You Are Your Child's First Teacher.* Berkeley: Celestial Arts, 1989.

Bell, Ruth. *Changing Bodies, Changing Lives.* New York: Vintage Books, 1987.

Bendall, Jean. *School's Out: Educating Your Child at Home.* Bath, England: Ashgrove Press, 1987.

Briggs, Anne. *Circumcision: What Every Parent Should Know.* Earlysville, Va.: Birth & Parenting Publications, 1984.

Britz-Crecelius, Heidi. *Children at Play: Preparation for Life.* New York: Inner Traditions International, 1972.

Colfax, David, and Micki Colfax. *Hard Times in Paradise.* New York: Warner Books, 1992.

_____. *Homeschooling for Excellence.* New York: Warner Books, 1988.

Coulter, Harris, and Barbara Fisher. *D.P.T.: A Shot in the Dark.* New York: Warner Books, 1985.

Cusick, Lois. *Waldorf Parenting Handbook.* New York: St. George Publications, 1984.

DeBold, Elizabeth, Marie Wilson, and Idelisse Malave. *Mother Daughter Revolution.* New York: Bantam Books, 1993.

Dreikurs, Rudolf. *Children the Challenge.* New York: Penguin, Plume, 1964.

Ebrahim, G. J. *Breastfeeding: The Biological Option.* New York: Pantheon Book/Schocken Books, 1978.

Faber, Adele, and E. Mazlish. *How to Talk So Kids Will Listen and Listen So Kids Will Talk.* New York: Avon Books, 1980.

_____. *Liberated Parents, Liberated Children.* N.p., n.d.

Halpern, Joshua. *Children of the Dawn: Visions of the New Family.* Bodega, Calif.: Only with Love Publications, 1986.

Hegener, Mark, and Helen Hegener. *The Homeschool Reader.* Tonasket, Wash.: Home Education Press, 1988.

Holt, John. *Teach Your Own.* New York: Dell Publishing, 1981.

_____. *Escape from Childhood.* New York: Elsevier Science Publishing, North-Holland, 1974.

_____. *How Children Learn.* New York: Pitman Publishing, 1967.

Kohn, Alfie. *Punished by Rewards.* New York: Houghton Mifflin, 1993.

Konner, Melvin. *Childhood.* Boston: Little, Brown, 1991.

La Leche League. *The Womanly Art of Breastfeeding.* New York: Penguin, Plume, 1981.

Liedloff, Jean. *The Continuum Concept.* Reading, Mass.: Addison-Wesley, 1985.

Lorie, Peter. *Wonder Child.* New York: Simon & Schuster, Fireside Books, 1989.

Martin, Richard. *A Parent's Guide to Childhood Symptoms.* New York: St. Martin's Press, 1982.

Mendelsohn, Robert. *How to Raise a Healthy Child in Spite of Your Doctor.* New York: Ballantine, 1984.

Montagu, Ashley. *Growing Young.* New York: McGraw-Hill, 1981.

Mothering Magazine. *Becoming a Father: Family, Work, and Self.* Santa Fe: John Muir Publications, 1990.

_____. *Immunizations.* Santa Fe: John Muir Publications, 1986.

Neill, A.S. *Summerhill: A Radical Approach to Childrearing.* New York: Hart Publishing, 1960.

Neustaedter, Randall. *The Immunization Decision: A Guide for Parents.* Berkeley: North Atlantic Books, 1990.

Rich, Adrienne. *Of Woman Born: Motherhood as Experience and Institution.* New York: W. W. Norton, 1986.

Rozman, Deborah. *Meditation for Children.* Boulder Creek, Calif.:University of the Trees Press, 1976.

Schultz, Karen. *A Theosophical Guide for Parents.* Ojai, Calif.: Parents Theosophical Research Group, 1984.

Thevenin, Tine. *The Family Bed: An Age Old Concept in Child Rearing.* Garden City, N.Y.: Avery Publishing Group, 1992.

Vissel, Joyce, and Barry Vissel. *Models of Love: The Parent-Child Journey.* Aptos, Calif. Ramira Publishing, 1986.

Wallerstein, Edward. *Circumcision: An American Health Fallacy.* NewYork: Springer Publishing, 1980.

West, Melissa G. *If Only I Were a Better Mother.* Walpole, N.H.: Stillpoint Publishing International, 1992.

Wootan, George. *Pediatrics: A Course for Parents.* Hurley, N.Y.: George Wootan, 1986.

❖ GENERAL HERBALISM ❖

Bear, Walking Night, and Stan Padilla. *Song of the Seven Herbs.* Summertown, Tenn.: Book Publishing, 1983.

Beinfield, Harriet, and Efrem Korngold. *Between Heaven and Earth: A Guide to Chinese Medicine.* New York: Ballantine, 1991.

Bennett, Jennifer. *Lilies of the Hearth.* Willowdale, Ontario: Camden House Publishing, 1991.

Birzneck, Ella. *Dominion Herbal College Manuals,* 3 vols. Burnaby, B.C.: Dominion Herbal College, 1962.

Conrow, Robert, and Arlene Hecksel. *Herbal Pathfinders.* Santa Barbara, Calif.: Woodbridge Press Publishing, 1983.

Cruden, Lorien. *Love Is Green: An Herbal for Parents.* Port Townsend, Wash.: Pan's Forest Herb Co., n.d.

Cummings, Stephen, and Dana Ullman. *Everybody's Guide to Homeopathic Medicines.* New York: St. Martin's Press, 1984.

de Bairacli-Levy, Juliette. *Nature's Children.* New York: Pantheon Books/ Schocken Books, 1971.

Dharmananda, Subhuti. *Chinese Herbology.* Portland: Institute for Traditional Medicine and Preventive Health Care, 1989.

_____. *Your Nature, Your Health: Chinese Herbs in Constitutional Therapy.* Portland: Institute for Traditional Medicine and Preventive Health Care, 1986.

Dodd, Deborah Lynn. *Non-Toxic and Natural.* New York: Jeremy P. Tarcher, 1985.

Frawley, David, and Vasant Lad. *The Yoga of Herbs.* Santa Fe: Lotus Press, 1986.

Gardner, Joy. *The New Healing Yourself.* Freedom, Calif.: The Crossing Press, 1989.

_____. *Healing Yourself During Pregnancy.* Freedom, Calif. : The Crossing Press, 1987.

_____. *Healing the Family.* New York: Bantam Books, 1982.

Grieve, Maude. *A Modern Herbal,* 2 vols. New York: Dover Publications, 1971.

Haas, Elson. *Staying Healthy with the Seasons.* Berkeley: Celestial Arts, 1981.

Hoffman, David. *The Holistic Herbal.* Forres, Scotland: Findhorn Press, 1983.

Hsu, Hong-yen. *Major Chinese Herbal Formulas.* Los Angeles: Oriental Healing Arts Institute, 1980.

Hylton, William, ed. *The Rodale Herb Book.* Emmaus, Pa.: Rodale Press, 1974.

Jackson, Mildred, and Terri Teague. *The Handbook of Alternatives to Chemical Medicine.* Oakland: Teague & Jackson, 1975.

King, Kurt. *Herbs to the Rescue: Herbal First Aid Handbook.* Hamilton, Mont.: Higher Ground Publications,1991.

Kloss, Jethro. *Back to Eden.* Loma Linda, Calif.: Back to Eden Books, 1981.

Kushi, Michio. *Macrobiotic Home Remedies.* New York: Japan Publications, 1985.

McIntyre, Anne. *The Herbal for Mother and Child.* Rockport, Mass.: Element, 1992.

Mowrey, Daniel. *The Scientific Validation of Herbal Medicine.* Cormorant Books, 1986.

Muramoto, Naboru. *Healing Ourselves.* New York: Avon Books, 1973.

Riggs, Maribeth. *Natural Child Care.* New York: Harmony Books, 1989.

Santillo, Humbart. *Natural Healing with Herbs.* Prescott Valley, Ariz.: Hohm Press, 1987.

Scott, Julian. *Natural Medicine for Children.* New York: Avon Books, 1990.

Slick, Rosemary Gladstar. *Herbs for Children.* East Barre, Vt.: Sage Healing Series, n.d.

Tierra, Lesley. *The Herbs of Life.* Freedom, Calif.: The Crossing Press, 1992.

Tierra, Michael. *Planetary Herbology.* Santa Fe: Lotus Press, 1988.

_____. *The Way of Herbs.* Santa Cruz: Orenda/Unity Press, 1980.

Veith, Ilza. *The Yellow Emperor's Classic of Internal Medicine.* Berkeley and Los Angeles: University of California Press, 1949.

Weed, Susun. *Healing Wise.* Woodstock, N.Y.: Ash Tree Publishing, 1989.

Wright, Machaelle. *Flower Essences.* Jeffersonton, Va.: Perelandra, 1988.

❖ FIELD GUIDES ❖

Audubon Society. *Field Guide to North American Trees.* New York: Alfred A. Knopf, 1980.

Elliot, Doug. *Woodslore and Wildwoods Wisdom.* Union Mills, N.C.: Possum Productions, 1986.

_____. *Roots: An Underground Botany and Forager's Guide.* Old Greenwich, Conn.: Chatham Press, 1976.

Foster, Steven, and James Duke. *Eastern/Central Medicinal Plants.* Boston: Houghton Mifflin, 1990.

Gabriel, Ingrid. *Herb Identifier and Handbook.* New York: Sterling Publishing, 1979.

Gibbons, Bob. *How Flowers Work: A Guide to Plant Botany.* Dorset, England: Blandford Press, 19484.

Gibbons, Euell. *Stalking the Healthful Herbs.* Putney, Vt.: Alan C. Hood, 1966.

Lee, Deborah. *Exploring Nature's Uncultivated Garden.* Takoma Park, Md.: Havelin Communications, 1989.

Meunick, Jim. *The Basic Essentials of Edible Wild Plants and Useful Herbs.* Merrillville, Ind.: ICS Books, 1988.

Moulton, Le Arta. *Herb Walk.* Provo: Gluten Co., 1979.

Peterson, Lee Allen. *A Field Guide to Wild Edible Plants, Eastern/Central.* Boston: Houghton Mifflin, 1977.

❖ CHILDBIRTH ❖

Arms, Suzanne. *Immaculate Deception.* New York: Bantam Books, 1975.

Baker, Jeannine P. "Deep Ecology of Birth." Monroe, Utah: Freestone Publishing, 1991.

Baker, Jeannine P., Frederick Baker, and Tamara Slaton. *Conscious Conception.* Sevier, Utah: Freestone Publishing, 1986.

Baldwin, Rahima. *Special Delivery.* Berkeley: Celestial Arts, 1986.

Corda, Murshida. *Cradle of Heaven: Psychological and Spiritual Dimensions of Conception, Pregnancy and Birth.* Lebanon Springs, N.Y.: Omega, 1987.

Dunham, Carroll. *Mamatoto: A Celebration of Birth.* New York: Penguin, Viking, 1991.

Flaws, Bob. *The Path of Pregnancy.* Boulder: Blue Poppy Enterprises Press, 1982.

Gaskin, Ina May. *Spiritual Midwifery.* Summertown, Tenn.: Book Publishing, 1980.

Goldsmith, Judith. *Childbirth Wisdom from the World's Oldest Societies.* New York: Congdon and Weed, 1984.

Hobbs, Valerie. *Herbs for Women: A Guide for Lay Midwives.* Valerie Hobbs, 1981; distributed by Cascade Health Care Products.

Huxley, Laura, and Piero Ferrucci. *The Child of Your Dreams.* Rochester, Vt.: Inner Traditions International, Destiny Books, 1992.

Kitzinger, Sheila. *The Complete Book of Pregnancy and Childbirth.* New York: Alfred A. Knopf, 1983.

_____. *Birth at Home.* New York: Penguin, 1979.

Klaus, Marshall, and John Kennell. *Bonding.* New York: Penguin, Plume, 1983.

Leboyer, Frederick. *The Art of Breathing.* Longmead, Great Britain: Element, 1983.

_____. *Inner Beauty, Inner Light: Yoga for Pregnant Women.* New York: Alfred A. Knopf, 1978.

Linden, Zur. *When a Child Is Born.* New York: Thorsens, 1984.

Mitford, Jessica. *The American Way of Birth.* New York: Penguin Books, Dutton, 1992.

Moskowitz, Richard. *Homeopathic Medicines for Pregnancy and Childbirth.* Berkeley: North Atlantic Press, 1992.

Noble, Elizabeth. *Childbirth with Insight.* Boston: Houghton Mifflin, 1983.

Panuthos, Claudia. *Transformation Through Birth.* South Hadley, Mass: Greenwood Publishing Group, Bergin & Garvey, 1984.

Peterson, Gayle. *Birthing Normally.* Berkeley: Mindbody Press, 1984.

Peterson, Gayle, and Lewis Mehl. *Pregnancy as Healing,* 2 vols. Berkeley: Mindbody Press, 1984.

Schwartz, Leni. *Bonding Before Birth.* Boston: Sigo Press, 1991.

Sears, William, and Martha Sears. *The Birth Book.* Boston: Little, Brown, 1994.

Weed, Susun. *Wise Woman Herbal for the Childbearing Year.* Woodstock, N.Y.: Ash Tree Publishing, 1985.

❖ NUTRITION AND COOKBOOKS ❖

Ballantine, Rudolph. *Diet and Nutrition.* Honesdale, Pa.: Himalayan Publishers, 1978.

Brewer, Gail S., and Tom Brewer. *What Every Pregnant Woman Should Know: The Truth about Diet and Drugs in Pregnancy.* New York: Penguin, 1977.

Colbin, Annemarie. *Food and Healing.* New York: Ballantine, 1986.

Dufty, William. *Sugar Blues.* New York: Warner Books, 1975.

Eisenberg, Arlene, Heidi E. Murkoff, and Sandee E. Hathaway. *What to Eat When You're Expecting.* New York: Workman Publishing, 1986.

Galland, Leo. *Superimmunity for Kids.* New York: Delta Books, 1988.

Garvey, John. *The Five Phases of Food.* Newtonville, Mass.: Wellbeing Books, 1985.

_____. *Yin and Yang: Two Hands Clapping.* Newtonville, Mass.: Wellbeing Books, 1985.

Kirschmann, John, and LaVonne Dunne. *Nutrition Almanac.* New York: McGraw-Hill, 1984.

Kushi, Michio, and Aveline Kushi. *Macrobiotic Pregnancy and Care of the Newborn.* New York: Japan Publications, 1983.

Luke, Barbara. *Maternal Nutrition.* Boston: Little, Brown, 1979.

Ni, Maoshing, and Cathy McNease. *The Tao of Nutrition.* Santa Monica: Shrine of the Eternal Breath of Tao, 1987.

Shandler, Michael, and Nina Shandler. *The Complete Guide and Cookbook for Raising Your Child as a Vegetarian.* New York: Ballantine, 1981.

❖ PHYSICAL EXERCISE, YOGA, MEDITATION, AND MASSAGE ❖

Baker, Jeannine P. *Prenatal Yoga and Natural Birth.* Berkeley: North Atlantic Press, 1986.

Carr, Rachel. *Be a Frog, a Bird, or a Tree.* New York: Harper & Row, 1973.

Cohen, Kenneth. *Imagine That: A Child's Guide to Yoga.* Santa Barbara: Santa Barbara Books, 1983.

Flaws, Bob. *Turtle Tail and Other Tender Mercies: Traditional Chinese Pediatrics.* Boulder: Blue Poppy Enterprises Press, 1985.

Markowitz, Elysa, and Howard Brainen. *Baby Dance: A Comprehensive Guide to Prenatal and Postpartum Exercise.* Englewood Cliffs, N.J.: Prentice Hall, 1980.

McClure, Vimala Schneider. *Infant Massage.* New York: Bantam Books, 1989.

Murdock, Maureen. *Spinning Inward: Using Guided Imagery with Children.* Boston: Shambhala Publications, 1987.

Rozman, Deborah. *Meditating with Children.* Boulder Creek, Calif.: University of the Trees Press, 1976.

❖ MEDICAL HISTORY ❖

Achterberg, Jeanne. *Woman as Healer.* Boston: Shambhala Publications, 1991.

Ehrenreich, Barbara, and Deidre English. *Witches, Midwives and Nurses: A History of Women Healers.* New York: Feminist Press at The City University of New York, 1973.

Grossinger, Richard. *Planet Medicine: From Stone Age Shamanism to Post-Industrial Healing.* Berkeley: North Atlantic Books, 1985.

Kaptchuk, Ted, and Michael Croucher. *The Healing Arts: Exploring the Medical Ways of the World.* New York: Simon & Schuster, Summit Books, 1987.

❖ POSITIVE ATTITUDE AND HEALING ❖

Grof, Stanislav. *The Holotropic Mind.* San Francisco: HarperCollins, 1990.

Hay, Louise. *You Can Heal Your Life.* Santa Monica: Hay House, 1984.

Marieschild, Diane. *Motherwit.* Freedom, Calif.: The Crossing Press, 1981.

Siegal, Bernie. *Peace, Love and Healing.* New York: Harper & Row, 1990.

❖ TEXTBOOKS AND TECHNICAL REFERENCE BOOKS ❖

Bates, Barbara. *A Guide to the Physical Examination,* 3d ed. Philadelphia: J. B. Lippincott, 1983.

Keay, A. J., and D. M. Morgan. *Craig's Care of the Newly Born Infant.* New York: Churchill Livingstone, 1982.

Tortora, Gerard, and Nicholas Anagnostakos. *Principles of Anatomy and Physiology.* New York: Harper & Row, 1984.

Werner, David. *Where There Is No Doctor: A Village Health-Care Handbook.* Palo Alto: Hesperian Foundation, 1977.

Index

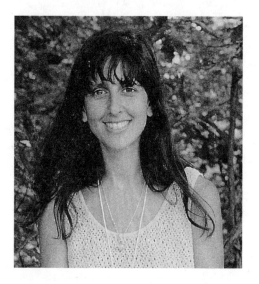

Since 1983 after leaving a pre-medical program at an early college for gifted teenagers, I have been a student and practitioner of family-centered natural health care. This path has led me to study independently through books, to study with many herbalists, to gain hands-on clinical experience, and to receive the necessary training to practice as a midwife. In addition, I have completed the requirements for Master Herbalist certification and have studied both western and eastern philosophies of health. I have found that natural remedies are not only generally safe, accessible, and affordable, but that they have brought my entire family closer to the natural world. While over ten years of midwifery and herbal practice has taught me a great deal about natural family health, my most profound teachers have been my husband and our four children, and the experiences we've had through times of both health and illness.

Aviva Romm

The Crossing Press
publishes many books on natural healing
for women, men and children.
To receive our current catalog,
please call toll-free,
800-777-1048.